Postnatal Care

**In Memoriam**

Dr Heather Winter very sadly died, aged 48, just after the final chapters for this book were finished. Heather had an important role in the production of this book and was pivotal in the research on postnatal care to which it was linked. Heather was qualified as an Obstetrician and Gynaecologist and a Public Health Doctor. She was a Senior Clinical Lecturer in Public Health and Epidemiology at Birmingham University, in which capacity she was an excellent teacher and researcher. Her main aim in life was to live and work in ways that could make a difference to the lives of others. In addition to her research on maternity care, she made major contributions in the areas of gynaecological cancer and in reduction of perinatal and maternal mortality in the developing world. Her contribution will be hugely missed by many.

*For Elsevier:*
*Commissioning Editor:* Mairi McCubbin
*Development Editor:* Sheila Black
*Project Manager:* Elouise Ball
*Designer:* Erik Bigland

# Postnatal Care
## Evidence and Guidelines for Management

SECOND EDITION

**Debra Bick**  BA MMedSci RGN RM

*Professor of Midwifery and Women's Health, Centre for Research in Midwifery and Childbirth, Faculty of Health and Human Sciences, Thames Valley University, London, UK*

**Christine MacArthur**  PhD

*Professor of Maternal and Child Epidemiology, Department of Public Health and Epidemiology, University of Birmingham, Edgbaston, Birmingham, UK*

**Heather Winter**  MD FRCOG MFPHM

*Senior Clinical Lecturer in Public Health and Epidemiology, Department of Public Health and Epidemiology, University of Birmingham, Edgbaston, Birmingham, UK*

With contributions from
Kathy de Mott and Gill Ritchie,
National Collaborating Centre for Primary Care, Royal College of General Practitioners

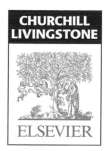

CHURCHILL LIVINGSTONE

ELSEVIER

EDINBURGH LONDON NEW YORK OXFORD PHILADELPHIA ST LOUIS SYDNEY TORONTO 2009

## CHURCHILL
## LIVINGSTONE
### ELSEVIER

An imprint of Elsevier Limited

© Elsevier Limited 2009. All rights reserved.

First published 2002
This edition 2009

ISBN 978-0-443-10400-8

**British Library Cataloguing in Publication Data**
A catalogue record for this book is available from the British Library

**Library of Congress Cataloging in Publication Data**
A catalog record for this book is available from the Library of Congress

**Notice**
Knowledge and best practice in this field are constantly changing. As new research and experience broaden our knowledge, changes in practice, treatment and drug therapy may become necessary or appropriate. Readers are advised to check the most current information provided (i) on procedures featured or (ii) by the manufacturer of each product to be administered, to verify the recommended dose or formula, the method and duration of administration, and contraindications. It is the responsibility of the practitioner, relying on their own experience and knowledge of the patient, to make diagnoses, to determine dosages and the best treatment for each individual patient, and to take all appropriate safety precautions.
To the fullest extent of the law, neither the Publisher nor the Authors assume any liability for any injury and/or damage to persons or property arising out of or related to any use of the material contained in this book.

The Publisher

**your source for books,
journals and multimedia
in the health sciences**

**www.elsevierhealth.com**

The publisher's policy is to use paper manufactured from sustainable forests

Printed in China

# Contents

# Preface

The evidence base and guidelines which form the main part of this book were originally developed as part of the IMPaCT (Implementing Midwifery-led Postnatal Care Trial) study (MacArthur et al 2002, 2003). The guidelines were developed as part of the new model of care, the main objective of which was to improve women's physical and psychological health after birth, through the systematic identification and management of their postpartum health problems. Postnatal midwifery care continued to be universally implemented as part of the new model. These guidelines were part of the new care package used by community midwives in the study to provide best evidence of effective management. As such, they were extensively reviewed and tested.

For the second edition, in order to ensure consistency with recently published guidance for postnatal care in England and Wales from the National Institute for Health and Clinical Excellence (NICE 2006), systematic reviews undertaken by the NICE guideline development team at the National Collaborating Centre for Primary Care (NCC-PC) have informed the update of evidence with respect to the identification and management of included health problems and symptoms. The guidelines were devised for use by practising midwives and assume a prior level of knowledge applicable to their training and experience, but will also be useful for other groups, such as midwifery and health visitor students, health visitors, family doctors and obstetricians, as well as women themselves. Although originally prepared for UK postnatal practice, the evidence presented is international and the guidelines are relevant to community-based care after childbirth in other countries in the developed world.

## Acknowledgements

This book was written in collaboration with the National Collaborating Centre for Primary Care. Dr Kathy de Mott and Gill Ritchie developed and implemented the search strategies for the systematic reviews which have informed the second edition.

Christine Henderson devised the original format of the accompanying leaflet sections for each guideline.

Debra Bick

*London and Birmingham, 2008*                                    Christine MacArthur

## References

MacArthur C, Winter H, Bick DE et al 2002 Effects of redesigned community postnatal care on women's health 4 months after birth: a cluster randomised controlled trial. Lancet 359: 378-385

MacArthur C, Winter HR, Bick DE et al 2003 Redesigning postnatal care; a randomised controlled trial of protocol based, midwifery led care focused on individual women's physical and psychological health needs. NHS Research and Development, NCC HTA, Southampton

National Institute for Health and Clinical Excellence (NICE) 2006 Postnatal care: routine postnatal care of women and their babies. Nice Clinical Guideline 37

# Introduction

The content of this book was originally derived from work undertaken for the IMPaCT study, a large cluster randomised controlled trial, funded by the NHS Research and Development Health Technology Assessment Programme, which compared a new model of midwifery-led postnatal care with current care (MacArthur et al 2002, 2003). The background to the IMPaCT study was informed by the recommendations of two major reports which sought to influence the direction of the maternity services in the 1990s: *Changing Childbirth*, the report of the Expert Committee on Maternity Care (Department of Health 1993), and the House of Commons Select Committee Report on the maternity services (House of Commons Health Committee 1992), and evidence from studies of maternal morbidity. These studies consistently found that women did not volunteer information about their health problems, but would provide information *if they were asked* (Bick & MacArthur 1995, Brown & Lumley 1998, Glazener et al 1995, MacArthur et al 1991). It was postulated that much morbidity remained unidentified because care continued to focus on routine observations and examinations, and that early discharge from midwifery care at around 10–14 days, together with a final postnatal consultation with the family doctor at 6 weeks, left insufficient time to adequately ascertain and manage women's health needs.

The new model of care which was developed, implemented and evaluated within the IMPaCT study required midwives to plan selective visits based on women's individual needs until 28 days rather than the usual 10–14 days. Symptom checklists were used to systematically identify health problems around the 10th and 28th days, and at a final consultation at around 10–12 weeks, which replaced the 6–8-week check with the family doctor. The Edinburgh Postnatal Depression Scale was also administered by the midwives at 28 days and 10–12 weeks to identify women who may have depression. The emphasis of the new model of care was on the identification and appropriate and timely management, including support and reassurance, of individual physical and psychological health needs. The evidence-based guidelines were developed to help achieve this. The results of the IMPaCT study showed that universal implementation of midwifery-led postnatal care, tailored to meet individual women's needs, made a significant difference to women's psychological health and well-being at 4 and 12 months after the birth, and more cost-effective use of healthcare resources (MacArthur et al 2002, 2003).

Since the publication of the first edition of this book and the results of the IMPaCT study, further major policy and practice initiatives have been published relevant to the provision and content of maternity care in England and Wales. In 2004, the National Service Framework for Children, Young People and Maternity Services (NSF) was published, one of the most complex and comprehensive publications relating to maternity and children's services to date, which aims to ensure that care from pregnancy and birth until a child reaches 18 years of age is informed by evidence-based quality standards. It includes a 10-year plan with explicit government support to improve the lives and health of children and young people. There are 11 core standards, including one for maternity care. Recommendations for postnatal care include that care from the midwife should be extended for all women until at least a month after the birth and for up to 3 months if appropriate; the provision of a community-based lead health professional (usually initially the midwife) to co-ordinate care following hospital discharge; and systematic identification and management of maternal health problems using a recognised assessment tool.

In 2006, the National Institute for Health and Clinical Excellence (NICE) published guidelines to inform the routine postnatal care a healthy woman and her baby should expect to receive from the NHS in England and Wales. The guideline includes recommendations which aim to assist healthcare professionals and women with the identification of signs and symptoms of major maternal and infant morbidity and common maternal and infant health problems. Guidance includes referral pathways, observations or examinations which should be undertaken within a specific time period to monitor recovery from birth or to comply with the national screening programme, and support for infant feeding. The guideline also recommends use of a care co-ordinator and 'signposts' use of a range of information for women and their families, including the *Birth to Five* publication. In 2007, NICE published a guideline on antenatal and postnatal mental health. The recommendations of these and other relevant NICE guidelines are reflected in the relevant chapters of this book.

The content and recommendations of the NICE postnatal care guideline considered evidence from the IMPaCT study (MacArthur et al 2002, 2003), including evidence relating to the identification of common maternal health problems, although guidance did not include recommendations for management beyond that deemed to fall within 'core' postnatal care. For example, it was beyond the remit of the guideline to include on the management of medical conditions recommendations experienced by a woman before, during or after her pregnancy, existing pregnancy-related and/or non-pregnancy related chronic or acute conditions or diseases, or any aspect of antepartum or intrapartum care.

When the authors were approached to produce a second edition of this book, consultation took place with members of the NCC-PC and the Guideline Development Group who were responsible for developing the recommendations for the NICE postnatal care guideline to produce a joint publication, given the need to ensure that recommendations for practice were consistent across the publications. Agreement was reached that the systematic reviews undertaken to inform the identification of common maternal health problems in the NICE guideline would be used to update the second edition of the book, with additional new reviews completed by the team from the NCC-PC to inform risk factors for the development of symptoms. The findings of the IMPaCT study, together with the recommendations of the NSF (Department of Health 2004) and the suite of NICE guidance relevant to maternity care (NICE 2006, 2007), have brought together evidence to ensure that all women receive care during the postnatal period which is timely and tailored to their individual need. Although NICE and DoH publications relate to maternity service policy, practice and service delivery in England and Wales, the book continues to present evidence and information of use nationally and internationally, which is why this second edition will continue to be of value for those who work with women and their infants after birth.

## DEVELOPMENT OF THE GUIDELINES

The procedure used to develop the guidelines was extensive, scientifically rigorous and took various stages, which are described briefly below. An example of the search strategies developed for the systematic reviews of the evidence is detailed in Appendix 1.

1. A systematic review of the literature was undertaken by members of the NCC-PC team on the health problems and symptoms which were the focus of the previous edition, many of which were also included in the NICE postnatal care guideline. The literature was searched to obtain an update of the evidence on the prevalence and risk factors of each problem area, using general population studies in the absence of specific postpartum studies. The same search strategies as used by the NCC-PC to develop the NICE postnatal care guideline were used, with additional strategies developed to inform areas excluded from the scope of the NICE guideline. The 'hierarchy of evidence' followed was that used by NICE (see Appendix 1).
2. Using the above information, each guideline update was then drafted by one of the authors.
3. The guidelines were then reviewed by other members of the editorial team, which includes expertise in midwifery, obstetrics and epidemiology, and revised as appropriate.

## HOW TO USE THE GUIDELINES

### Format of the guidelines

Each guideline has three sections as described below.

*Section one:* this presents the **full review of evidence** relating to each health problem or symptom, including definition, frequency of occurrence, risk factors and management. The evidence presented, although focused on primary management, sometimes includes evidence on secondary management, in order that a comprehensive picture is made available.

*Section two:* this consists of a much briefer and more practical '**What to Do'** section. It summarises the evidence in the form of advice on best practice, always including clear criteria referral. The priority levels for referral follow those included in the NICE postnatal care guideline (NICE 2006) shown below, but clinical judgement should be used at all times.

| Status | Classification |
|---|---|
| Emergency | Life-threatening or potentially life-threatening condition |
| Urgent | Potentially serious situation, which needs appropriate action |
| Non-urgent | Continue to monitor and assess |

NICE (2006), p.41

*Section three:* this comprises a **leaflet** version based on the 'What to Do' section but presented in an even briefer format. The leaflets were developed to be easily carried around by healthcare professionals.

### How to read the guidelines

Section one of each guideline should be read in full at some time, to enable familiarity with the complete evidence base for the management advice given in sections two and three. However, recognising that workload and other circumstances will not always allow the opportunity to read and fully digest this detailed information prior to use, all the sections, as well as each guideline, have been written to 'stand alone'. This facilitates pragmatic use, although those who do read from beginning to end will find some repetition, in particular, in describing studies that are applicable to more than one guideline area.

### WHEN TO USE THE GUIDELINES

The guidelines were originally developed for use in the IMPaCT study throughout the whole period of postnatal community midwifery contact, which was up to 3 months postpartum, although much of the information is likely to be applicable for longer. Some guidelines, however, are more likely to be used during the first few days (for example, uterine infection and abnormal bleeding, abdominal wound care) and others at later visits (for example, depression, backache, fatigue).

## SYMPTOM IDENTIFICATION CHECKLIST

The guidelines are appropriate when health problems or symptoms are identified, which can be by the healthcare professional observing a problem or the woman (or her partner or family) reporting it. One of the findings of the postpartum morbidity studies, however, was that many health problems had not been reported to the relevant professionals. In order to ensure systematic identification of problems, a symptom checklist was used by the midwives in the IMPaCT trial. This was used on about the 10th and 28th postnatal day and at the 10–12-week final consultation, although it would be appropriate for use at other times. A copy of this checklist is included in Appendix 2.

## References

Bick DE, MacArthur C 1995 Attendance, content and relevance of the six week postnatal examination. Midwifery 11:69-73

Brown S, Lumley J 1998 Maternal health after childbirth: results of an Australian population based survey. Br J Obstet Gynaecol 105:156-161

Department of Health 1993 Changing childbirth. The report of the Expert Maternity Group. HMSO, London

Department of Health 2004 National service framework for children, young people and maternity services. Stationery Office, London

Glazener C, Abdalla M, Stroud P 1995 Postnatal maternal morbidity: extent, causes, prevention and treatment. Br J Obstet Gynaecol 102:282-287

House of Commons Health Committee 1992 Report on the maternity services, volume 1. Stationery Office, London

MacArthur C, Lewis M, Knox E 1991 Health after childbirth. HMSO, London

MacArthur C, Winter H, Bick DE et al 2002 Effects of redesigned community postnatal care on women's health 4 months after birth: a cluster randomised controlled trial. Lancet 359:378-385

MacArthur C, Winter HR, Bick DE et al 2003 Redesigning postnatal care; a randomised controlled trial of protocol based, midwifery led care focused on individual women's physical and psychological health needs. NHS Research and Development, NCC HTA, Southampton

National Institute for Health and Clinical Excellence (NICE) 2006 Postnatal care: routine postnatal care of women and their babies. Nice Clinical Guideline 37

National Institute for Health and Clinical Excellence (NICE) 2007 Antenatal and postnatal mental health: clinical management and service guidance. NICE Clinical Guideline 45

# Chapter 1

# Endometritis and abnormal blood loss

## INTRODUCTION

Of the half million maternal deaths worldwide each year, 99.5% of which occur in developing countries, haemorrhage remains the leading cause, with deaths due to sepsis estimated at 79,000 (15%) (AbouZahr & Wardlaw 2004, Khan et al 2006). The introduction of antibiotics during the interwar years, alongside changes in obstetric care, contributed to a reduction in levels of maternal mortality and morbidity from puerperal infection and postpartum haemorrhage. Health professionals with responsibility for postnatal care are being urged to continue to be vigilant to the development of puerperal infection; 16 maternal deaths as a direct consequence of puerperal sepsis were recorded during the triennial period 2003–2005 (Lewis 2007). Less severe cases can contribute to the high level of morbidity generally experienced by women following childbirth (Glazener et al 1995, MacArthur et al 1991). Traditionally midwifery postnatal care has included routine assessment of temperature, uterine involution and observation of lochia to detect deviations from normal physiological recovery following childbirth. The value of such routine assessments by midwives has been questioned in recent years (Marchant et al 1996).

The source of puerperal sepsis is likely to be the genital tract but the term would embrace any cause of sepsis in the puerperium. The terms genital tract sepsis, uterine infection and endometritis are also used, almost interchangeably throughout the literature. We have used endometritis.

Postpartum haemorrhage (PPH) is classified as primary when it occurs within 24 hours of the birth and secondary thereafter (WHO 2003). Postpartum haemorrhage can be catastrophic at any stage of the puerperium, but routine postnatal care usually relates to determining whether a woman's vaginal loss after the first 24 hours constitutes abnormal bleeding and this is the term used here.

The exact nature of the link between abnormal bleeding and uterine infection or endometritis is not clear. Endometritis may be at the root of all cases of abnormal bleeding, as even minor 'retained' products of conception or intrapartum contamination may form a focus of infection. In some cases suspected sepsis is the predominant feature, while in others abnormal bleeding may occur in the absence of any evidence of sepsis. Therefore, abnormal bleeding and endometritis are considered separately in this guideline but, given their interrelationship, crossover is inevitable and their management is considered together.

## ENDOMETRITIS

### Definition

Endometritis occurs as a result of contamination of the endometrial cavity with vaginal organisms during labour and delivery. Invasion of the myometrium may occur and the highly vascular environment of the postpartum genital tract predisposes to the development of septicaemia. This can be rapid and overwhelming and 'puerperal fever' was and, as described above, in developing countries still is, an important cause of maternal death. Infection can impede the natural process of uterine involution and lead to severe postpartum haemorrhage. Therefore, if not identified and managed early, high rates of morbidity and even mortality can occur.

A standard definition of endometritis or uterine infection was not found. The causal organisms are usually normal inhabitants of the genital tract (Pastorek & Sanders 1991) and gaining a sample for culture without contamination is problematic, so positive culture is not a prerequisite for diagnosis. In the past, midwifery rules and codes of practice regulated care by defining the range of temperature rise which would initiate referral to a medical practitioner. For example, the Central Midwives Board Rules of 1962 stated that if a woman had 'a rise of temperature above 99.4° F, on three successive days, or a rise of temperature to 100.4° F, a registered medical practitioner must be summoned' (p. 60). With subsequent revisions to these rules and codes over the last four decades, there is no longer a defined range for what constitutes pyrexia. A transient elevation in maternal temperature is not uncommon during the postnatal period, for example among women who experience breast engorgement on or about the third postpartum day (RCM 2002), although the aetiology of this is unclear. The genital tract is a primary source of infection at this time, although other sites of infection must be considered (Calhoun & Brost 1995).

The World Health Organization (WHO) identifies the symptoms of uterine infection as a temperature >38° C and any of the following: feeling very weak, abdominal tenderness, foul-smelling lochia, profuse lochia, uterus not well contracted, lower abdominal pain or history of heavy vaginal bleeding (WHO 2006).

The threshold for treating as endometritis a pyrexial postpartum woman in whom alternative sources of infection have been excluded is likely to vary both individually and institutionally. In one study (Parrot et al 1989), irrespective of cause being established, antibiotics were prescribed for all women with a temperature of 37.8° C for more than 24 hours after a caesarean section. NICE guidelines state that sepsis may be suspected in the presence of **two or more of these signs and symptoms**: fever >38.5° C on one occasion or fever of 38° C taken 4 hours apart; chills; abdominal tenderness and no other recognised source of infection; uterine subinvolution; offensive or heavy lochia or tachycardia (NICE 2006). The level of evidence for this recommendation is a best practice point based on the experience of the Guideline Development Group.

In practice, however, endometritis is effectively the default diagnosis for any febrile illness without other cause in the immediate postpartum period, especially within the first 24 hours.

## Frequency of occurrence

Lack of a standard definition makes it difficult to ascertain accurate rates of occurrence and the estimate will be affected by the rigour with which alternative sources of infection are sought in pyrexial postpartum women, and by the level of ascertainment of infection after discharge from hospital.

In a random sample of women delivered vaginally at an Iowa hospital over a 14 -year period, the rate of endometritis was 1.6% (Ely et al 1996), and a study from Israel of the outcome of 75,947 term and preterm singleton deliveries between 1980 and 1997 found an endometritis rate of 0.17% following vaginal delivery and 2.63% following caesarean section (Chaim et al 2000). With retrospective reviews, however, it is difficult to be sure that follow-up was complete as women with endometritis may not be readmitted or may be admitted to a different unit. Using routine health insurer data, Yokoe et al (2001) estimated rates of endometritis at 0.2% following vaginal delivery and 0.8% after caesarean section during the first 30 days postpartum. As with other postpartum infections, estimates of occurrence of endometritis are now influenced by the use of prophylactic antibiotics, particularly following caesarean section.

Findings from the BLiPP study (Alexander et al 1997), described in more detail below, suggest that approximately 2% of women are admitted to hospital with complications associated with abnormal vaginal bleeding and/or uterine infection within 12 weeks of delivery.

## Risk factors

The most important risk factor for endometritis is caesarean delivery. Smaill & Hofmeyr (2000) reviewed 66 trials of antibiotic prophylaxis in caesarean section. Endometritis was consistently classified across trials as pyrexia in the absence of another cause. In the control groups, the overall incidence of endometritis in women undergoing elective caesarean section was 6.4% and 28.6% in women who had an emergency caesarean. The use of antibiotic prophylaxis for both planned and unplanned caesarean had a significant protective effect against endometritis, reducing the rate of endometritis by two-thirds.

Other factors reported to predispose to endometritis after vaginal deliveries, as presented in the background to a protocol for a Cochrane systematic review of treatment regimes, include: bacterial vaginosis; genital cultures positive for anaerobic gram-negative bacilli; prolonged rupture of the membranes; the presence of meconium during labour; low infant birth weight and multiple vaginal examinations (French & Smaill 2004). No association between postnatal endometritis and the use of water for pain relief or delivery has been found (Robertson et al 1998).

## ABNORMAL BLOOD LOSS

The main terms used to define abnormality in relation to postpartum vaginal loss are abnormal bleeding and secondary postpartum haemorrhage.

## Abnormal bleeding

Textbooks of midwifery and obstetrics suggest that the postpartum vaginal loss should no longer be red after the first 7 days and lochia should diminish within 4–8 weeks of delivery (Abbott et al 1997, Howie 1986). This definition of normal postnatal vaginal loss formed the basis for practice, and any deviation from it would be defined as abnormal bleeding. However, the evidence base for these assumptions is not described and evidence from more recent studies suggests that the normal duration and character of vaginal loss postpartum may be much more varied (Marchant et al 1999, Oppenheimer et al 1986, Visness et al 1997).

Oppenheimer et al (1986), in a prospective cohort study, recruited 617 women who delivered a live infant during a 10-week period and interviewed them within 48 hours of delivery. Each was asked to complete a diary sheet for up to 60 days and record one of three categories (lochia rubra, serosa and alba) which best described the colour of their lochia. Women were also given a fourth choice to describe when vaginal loss had ceased or normal pre-pregnancy discharge returned. Diary sheets were returned when no loss had been recorded for 7 days, except for recurrence of menses; only 236 women (38%) completed and returned diary sheets. The median duration of lochia rubra was 4 days and for lochia serosa, 22 days; 87 (36%) women did not experience lochia alba, as their loss ceased with lochia serosa. No mean duration of lochia alba was given for the remaining 149 women. Results confirmed clinical impressions that lochia persists for longer than is generally anticipated; 15% of women still had lochia serosa at 6 weeks postpartum, and 4% at 60 days. The researchers concluded that prolonged vaginal loss was neither unusual or abnormal, although some caution should be applied to these findings because of the low response rate.

Visness et al (1997) carried out a prospective study of breastfeeding women in Manila, The Philippines, to examine their experience of postnatal vaginal loss and compare findings with the duration and stages of lochia, as described in a commonly used obstetric text book in the USA. The study was undertaken as part of a randomised controlled trial of the effectiveness of the lactational amenorrhoea method of contraception. All women who chose this method of contraception, had given birth vaginally and had previously breastfed a child for a minimum of 12 months were invited to take part; 477 consented (the total number of eligible women was not given). Follow-up was for 1 year from the day of delivery. The women were given calendars to record daily, starting from the day of delivery, whether they had experienced vaginal bleeding or spotting. The median duration of lochia was 27 days (range 5–90 days) and did not vary by age, parity, infant characteristics or breastfeeding frequency. A quarter of the women reported that blood loss stopped and then recommenced. Lochia lasted for longer than the period of 2 weeks defined in the obstetric textbook and the return of menses was rare before 8 weeks.

It would be difficult to replicate this study in the UK, as few women continue breastfeeding beyond 6 months (Bolling et al 2007) and those that do are likely to have sociodemographic characteristics which differ from the general childbearing population. However, that lochial flow persisted up to and beyond the sixth postnatal week was confirmed by a UK study – the Blood Loss in the Postnatal Period (BLiPP) study (Marchant et al 1999). BLiPP was a three-part research study to investigate the hypothesis that 'routine abdominal palpation of uterine fundal height in postnatal women from 24 hours after delivery until the midwife discharges the woman from her care, fails to predict abnormal uterine bleeding or uterine infection' (Marchant & Alexander 1996, p. 402). One aim of the first part of the study was to describe the range of normal vaginal loss from 24 hours until 3 months after delivery.

To collect data for this, a prospective survey of 524 women from two health districts in the south of England was carried out between 1995 and 1996. Women were asked to complete two questionnaires and two diaries at intervals up to 16 weeks post delivery. Information on demographic and delivery characteristics were obtained from birth registers for all eligible women (i.e. women who delivered in the local area and who could speak/read/write English). The first questionnaire was completed from 48 hours to 5 days after delivery, depending on whether study recruitment had taken place on the postnatal ward or if the woman had been contacted following discharge. Women were asked about their experience of vaginal loss immediately following delivery and about the loss experienced on the day the questionnaire was completed. They were offered a range of descriptions to help them answer questions on the colour and amount of vaginal loss; 350 (67%) women responded. Between days 2 and 10, women completed the first diary (318 (61%) responded), followed by the second diary completed on the 14th, 21st and 28th postnatal days (284 (54%) responded). Women were asked to record details about various aspects of their postnatal health, such as psychological state and infant feeding, as well as the amount and duration of vaginal loss. The second questionnaire, sent 3 months after delivery, included questions on the duration and description of vaginal loss and about any problems associated with prolonged or excessive vaginal loss after the first 28 days up to completion of the questionnaire; 324 (62%) women responded.

Vaginal loss was more varied in the amount, colour and duration than described in commonly used midwifery textbooks, a similar finding to that of Visness et al (1997). The duration of vaginal loss ranged from 2 to 86 days after delivery, with a mean of 24 days. Duration was not associated with parity and 6% of women reported vaginal loss from 6 weeks up to 12 weeks postpartum. One interesting finding was that seven (4%) of the 175 primiparae who returned the first questionnaire were unaware that they would experience blood loss after childbirth. Of the 324 women who returned the questionnaire, 64 (20%) had been worried about their vaginal loss between 28 days and 3 months following the birth (Marchant et al 2002). The most common problems reported were passage of clots and heavy or moderate loss. The researchers concluded that findings could be used to inform women and health professionals of the colour, amount and duration of vaginal loss for the first 3 months following childbirth.

## Secondary postpartum haemorrhage (PPH)

Secondary PPH has traditionally been defined as a severe blood loss occurring after the first 24 hours of delivery and up to 6 weeks postpartum. Alternative definitions of secondary PPH vary in the time since birth (Alexander et al 2003) or in not defining any interval as being postpartum (Schuurmans et al 2000, WHO 2003). NICE postnatal guidelines have defined primary and secondary PPH as excessive vaginal blood loss but there is no precise definition of what constitutes a severe or excessive blood loss (NICE 2006). That bleeding is 'severe' will sometimes be self-evident, but is mostly subjective at the point where advice is sought. In clinical practice the passage of 'large' blood clots is often used as an indication of potential problems. There is no evidence base to show if the size or number of clots passed is indicative of potential or actual morbidity. In the absence of relevant evidence the decision to take further action will continue to be subjective.

## Frequency of occurrence

Because the definition of 'severe blood loss' is imprecise, the incidence of secondary PPH is difficult to ascertain, as reports may only refer to the most adverse outcomes. Prospective studies were not found and, as with endometritis, retrospective hospital-based reviews are likely to be underestimates as patients managed in the community and those admitted to other units will not be included. In one such case-note review in Hong Kong, the secondary PPH cases identified formed 0.38% of all deliveries, but the authors gave no details on how complete ascertainment of cases was likely to have been (Fung et al 1996). The rate of secondary PPH cases over a 2-year period between 1978 and 1980 in Detroit was 1.5%, but again no assessment can be made of case ascertainment for this study (Lee et al 1981). Rome (1975) estimated the rate of occurrence in his series to be 1.3%. As reported under endometritis, approximately 2% of women are admitted to hospital with complications associated with abnormal vaginal bleeding and/or uterine infection within 12 weeks of delivery (Alexander et al 1997).

## Risk factors

The International Federation of Gynecology and Obstetrics reported the most common causes of secondary PPH to be subinvolution of the placental site, infection and retained products of conception (RPOC) (ACOG 1990). Retained products of conception may provide the focus for infection or their presence may mechanically inhibit retraction of the uterus. RPOC were found in 17.9% of 106 women with secondary PPH in Rome's (1975) series.

It is likely, however, that excessive bleeding will not always occur with retained products of conception and an ultrasound study supports this (Tekay & Joupila 1993). In some cases of secondary PPH, the primary problem may be failure of the normal process of involution without either infection or RPOC.

Khong & Khong (1993) undertook a case-note and histological review of women with postpartum haemorrhage occurring between 24 hours and 6 months following delivery. The purpose of the study was to look for evidence of abnormal placentation in women who had secondary postpartum haemorrhage. In the non-pregnant uterus, the arteries are small in diameter and spiral. In the process of forming the placental bed in pregnancy, these vessels become much larger and more flaccid. Failure of this normal placentation has been linked with fetal growth retardation, pre-eclampsia and other pregnancy conditions (Khong et al 1986, Pijnenborg et al 1991). The authors' aim was to determine evidence of failure of the normal process whereby these vessels collapse and thrombose prior to regeneration of the normal non-pregnant pattern. They called this subinvolution of the placental bed.

The study population was defined by histological material received by the pathology laboratory at one Australian hospital. Therefore, women who were managed conservatively or had surgery but from whom no material was obtained were excluded. Of the 169 cases identified over a 5-year period between 1986 and 1991, 109 (64.5%) presented within 6 weeks of delivery and 54 (35.5%) between 6 weeks and 6 months postpartum. Including cases up to 6 months later in the analysis means the findings could relate to a subsequent pregnancy, and the following results relate to the cases presenting within 6 weeks. In 32% (n = 35) of the 109 cases presenting before 6 weeks, retained placental tissue was identified. Evidence of endometritis was adjudged to be present in only 4.6% (n = 5). The authors classified 20.2% (n = 22) as showing 'subinvolution of placental bed vessels', the remaining 43.1% (n = 47) specimens being 'non-diagnostic material', normal endometrium, decidua or showed 'normal' placental involution.

The study also attempted to explore associations between this finding and the conditions associated with abnormal placentation during pregnancy. Review of the clinical case notes was undertaken but no associations were found.

## Uterine involution

In addition to charting postpartum vaginal loss and measuring temperature in an attempt to detect and treat endometritis and secondary postpartum haemorrhage early, much of women's routine postpartum care has been centred on the measurement of uterine involution. Whether failure of involution is a risk factor or an effect of endometritis and postpartum haemorrhage is not clear, but its importance and detection are considered here.

Involution describes the return of the uterus to a pelvic position and the progress of involution is usually assessed by measurement of the symphysio-fundal distance (S-FD). This is the distance from the top of the uterine fundus to the top of the symphysis pubis. Delayed uterine involution is referred to as subinvolution of the uterus and is diagnosed by perceived delay in the reduction of the size of the uterus. There is limited information about the number of women diagnosed as having subinvolution, the relationship between subinvolution alone and subsequent outcome, the referral rate and the most appropriate management of subinvolution as a solitary sign.

The methods most commonly used to assess involution are anthropometry (simple abdominal palpation) or a tape measure. Midwifery textbooks vary in their description of the rate at which uterine involution occurs and lack detail of how the measurement of fundal height should be obtained (Cluett et al 1995). Nevertheless, failure of the uterus to involute could indicate the presence of retained products of conception. One study, undertaken to describe uterine involution in a small sample of primiparae who had a normal vaginal delivery (n = 28), found considerable variability in the pattern of uterine involution, not only between women but also in the daily rate of decline experienced by individual women (Cluett et al 1997). Twenty-two women had at least one episode of 'slow decline' (defined as a decline in the

S-FD of <1 cm over three or more days) at various times during the puerperium. It is possible that variability in the pattern of decline could be even greater amongst multiparae and those who had a caesarean section.

Because there was no evidence to suggest that midwives could measure S-FD with precision, Cluett et al (1995) investigated intraobserver variability, where the same midwife measured the same women using a tape measure, and interobserver variability, where different midwives measured the same women. Results showed that there was a significant degree of error in measurement of the S-FD when measurements for the same women were taken repeatedly by the same midwife, and the degree of error was even greater when measurements from the same women were taken by different midwives. The disparity between the inter- and intrarater observations suggests that measurement of uterine involution is unreliable. The authors concluded that measuring S-FD with a tape measure is not precise enough to enable clinical judgements to be made about normal or abnormal progress of uterine involution, and should be discontinued.

An earlier case control study also assessed the value of the postpartum measurement of the S-FD. Bergstrom & Libombo (1992) compared one group of 51 women who had clinically evident signs of endometritis-myometritis with 51 women matched for age, parity and number of days postpartum who had no signs of infection. They found that there was no significant difference between the S-FD measurements between the two groups. These researchers concluded that an infected uterus does not differ in fundal height from a healthy uterus. However, the findings should be interpreted with caution, as the study did not assess the level of accuracy of measurements obtained and the controls were matched only to within 2 postpartum days.

On the basis of these findings, NICE (2006) has concluded that there is no evidence to support the routine measurement of fundal height or how often uterine assessment should be undertaken. NICE (2006) has also stated that the evidence does not identify an accurate method to measure vaginal loss, and that there is no reliable evidence that uterine assessment alone is of value. The guideline does, however, point out that uterine assessment can be used to discount or confirm morbidity in combination with other symptoms such as fever, uterine or abdominal tenderness. The level of evidence for these recommendations is often the least optimal, however – a recommendation for best practice based on the experience of the Guideline Development Group. Better evidence is needed to inform this area of care.

## INVESTIGATION AND MANAGEMENT OF SUSPECTED ENDOMETRITIS OR ABNORMAL BLOOD LOSS

Routine measurement of the uterus may have little value, but its assessment in the context of other factors, such as the presence of abdominal tenderness, pyrexia, offensive lochia and a change in the nature and amount of lochia, may help establish a diagnosis of endometritis.

## Investigation

Some women with abnormal bleeding or suspected uterine infection will require investigation and will be referred for an ultrasound scan. As a result of the scan findings, the woman may undergo evacuation to remove retained products of conception. No controlled trials have been undertaken of the routine use of ultrasound to diagnose accurately the complications of involution or prolonged bleeding (Montgomery & Alexander 1994). Hertzberg & Bowie (1991) reviewed the ultrasound images of 53 postnatal women referred for possible retained products. Ultrasound findings were correlated with clinical and pathological reports on women who underwent an evacuation of retained products of conception (ERPC). Only 11 of 53 women had pathologically proven retained placental tissue. The most common finding in women with confirmed pathology was an echogenic mass in the uterine cavity (n = 9). These authors noted that the interpretation of ultrasound findings should be undertaken by an expert prior to performing curettage.

Studies have shown that, in some cases, debris in the uterine cavity may be normal in the early postnatal period. Tekay & Joupila (1993) carried out a longitudinal study to investigate postnatal alterations in peripheral vascular resistance of uterine arteries. Repeat ultrasound observations were performed on 42 postnatal women who had no symptoms of abnormal bleeding. One finding was the detection of debris in the uterine cavity in 21% of women during the first postpartum week, none of whom experienced subsequent morbidity.

As part of a study which evaluated ultrasound assessment of the uterine cavity postpartum, Carlan et al (1997) scanned 131 women immediately after the placenta was delivered. The 131 women then had their uterus explored manually and with sponge curettage. With a sensitivity for ultrasound of only 44% in detecting RPOC, the authors had to conclude that the appearance of retained products immediately after placental delivery is very variable.

## Management

In cases where women are pyrexial, may or may not have excessive blood loss but have other clinical symptoms (pyrexia, offensive lochia, uterine tenderness), antibiotics are usually prescribed and the symptoms managed conservatively. The choice of antibiotic regimen is usually empirical, with a spectrum of coverage which will eradicate the mixture of anaerobic and aerobic organisms potentially involved. The effect of different antibiotic regimens for the treatment of postpartum endometritis on failure of therapy and complications was systematically reviewed (French & Smaill 2004). The review identified 39 studies involving 4221 women, although overall they were not methodologically strong and often funded by the drug companies. The authors concluded that the combination of gentamicin and clindamycin is appropriate for the treatment of endometritis, that regimens with activity against penicillin-resistant anaerobic bacteria are better than those without and that there is no evidence that any one regimen is associated with fewer side-effects. Once uncomplicated endometritis has clinically improved with intravenous therapy, oral therapy is not needed.

For cases of secondary postpartum haemorrhage where bleeding is obviously severe, resuscitation and admission to hospital are required. If findings suggestive of subinvolution or endometritis are accompanied by moderate or prolonged haemorrhage, surgical intervention to perform uterine curettage continues to be a common method of management.

The need to perform surgery on all women who present with secondary PPH has, however, been questioned. Fung and colleagues (1996) conducted a retrospective case-note analysis at a hospital in Hong Kong to record the clinical features of 78 women diagnosed over a 3-year period with secondary PPH. No details were given of how long after delivery a diagnosis of secondary PPH was made. Thirty-one women (40%) were treated conservatively with antibiotics and all made a good recovery: 47 (60%) had surgical intervention but in only 23 cases were retained products found on histology. The authors concluded that half of the women did not require surgery, with caesarean section and a history of pyrexia being the only useful indicators in deciding whether to undertake surgical intervention – both being suggestive that conservative management should be used. Other observations made included a lack of correlation between the severity and timing of the bleeding and retained products. The authors concluded that further prospective studies are required to test the validity of their findings.

## SUMMARY OF THE EVIDENCE USED IN THIS GUIDELINE

- Endometritis should continue to be considered in all women with a postpartum pyrexia, especially if delivery was by caesarean section.
- Observational studies have shown more normal variation in the pattern of postpartum vaginal loss than previously described.
- There is no precise definition of what constitutes abnormal bleeding nor what amounts to severe blood loss and, therefore, secondary PPH.
- The evidence does not identify an accurate method to measure vaginal loss.
- There is no evidence to support the routine measurement of fundal height or how often uterine assessment should be undertaken.
- There is no reliable evidence that uterine assessment alone is of value, but NICE guidelines state that it can be used to discount or confirm morbidity in combination with other symptoms such as fever or abdominal tenderness.
- Ultrasound studies have shown apparent retained products of conception in women who have not experienced problems with excessive bleeding or infection. Further studies are required to ascertain the benefit of ultrasound to detect complications of involution or prolonged bleeding.

- One retrospective case-note analysis found that conservative management of secondary PPH was appropriate in at least half of the presenting cases. Further prospective studies are required to determine optimal management.

## WHAT TO DO

### Initial assessment – All women

- From delivery details note any problems with delivery or completeness of the third stage. Obtain a 'baseline' evaluation of the uterus (the uterus should be well contracted, non-tender and central). Explain what you are doing and why, encouraging the woman to feel her uterus to increase awareness of body changes during the puerperium. Ask her to describe the pattern of her loss since delivery. Note date and result of last Hb estimate. Personal hygiene should be discussed as appropriate. It may be helpful to explain that maternity-size pads should be used and to give an estimate of how often these should be changed.
- Assess blood loss. Advise that the amount of loss may be heavy during the first few days, but will gradually become less. The duration of lochia may vary. Lochia should have a non-offensive odour.
- Advise the woman to contact her midwife if she has a recurrence of bright red fresh loss after the first postpartum week or passes a large blood clot on more than one occasion.
- Women who report a heavier blood loss after breastfeeding should be reassured that this is normal, provided the loss subsides thereafter. Women who report lower abdominal pains suggestive of uterine origin at any time during the postnatal period and who are not breastfeeding should be monitored.

### Other visits

- Ask the woman specifically about her observation of lochia. Other indications (i.e. amount and colour of blood loss, offensive lochia, abdominal tenderness, general malaise, fever) should be taken into account before deciding if uterine palpation is required.
- Whatever non-barrier method of contraception a woman decides to use, information about the method should also include a description of possible side-effects, including vaginal loss or spotting.
- NICE guidelines (NICE 2006) recommend that all women should be advised to report to a healthcare professional any vaginal loss that does not stop by the sixth week after birth.
- NICE guidelines (NICE 2006) recommend, as a good practice point, that if a woman has sustained a postpartum haemorrhage or is experiencing persistent fatigue, her haemoglobin level should be evaluated and if low, treated according to local policy.

## Deviation from anticipated normal recovery

### Abnormal blood loss

- Ask the woman when she became concerned about her loss and how frequently pads have required changing (were they soaked or moderately stained? Ask for a quantifiable description of loss, e.g. 3 inch stain). Ascertain thickness of pads used. Ask her to describe the colour of loss, i.e. was it bright red, dark, medium or light red, or pale pink? Observe loss on the pad the woman is currently wearing. If the woman has passed large clots these should be examined for RPOC. Is the loss offensive now or has it been offensive?
- Did loss occur following a particular activity, i.e. breastfeeding? A heavier blood loss can be associated with some activities – reassure.
- Perform abdominal palpation and check temperature if loss is unrelated to other activities. If the uterus is central and well contracted, reassure and advise the woman to continue to observe lochia.
- If the uterus feels tender but loss is no longer heavy, arrange to visit the following day to assess condition. Advise that if bleeding is excessive in the meantime, the woman must contact her healthcare professional.
- If the uterus is tender and/or the loss is heavy, check temperature, take HVS and refer (urgent action). A dipstix analysis of urine should also be performed prior to referral, to exclude the possibility of a UTI (refer to guideline on Urinary Problems).
- If a woman continues to have prolonged heavy blood loss (more than a heavy period) but no evidence of infection or subinvolution, she should be asked at subsequent visits about her general well-being. It may be helpful to check her last Hb result. A woman who is symptomatic of anaemia should be referred.

### Offensive lochia (women will generally refer to this as blood loss)

- Confirm lochia are offensive. Is the colour of the lochia different from previously? Have any blood clots been passed? Exclude infected perineal wound or poor personal hygiene.
- Check the woman's temperature and gently palpate her abdomen. If she is pyrexial and/or has severe abdominal or pelvic pain, take HVS and dipstix analysis of urine and refer immediately (emergency action). This action should be taken even if other observations are within expected normal range, but her lochia are offensive.

### Pyrexia (temperature >38°C)

- If a woman is unwell, take her temperature. NICE guidelines state sepsis may be suspected in the presence of two or more of these signs and symptoms: temperature >38.5°C on one occasion or >38°C on two occasions 4 hours apart; with sign or symptoms which could include chills; abdominal tenderness and no other recognised source of infection; uterine subinvolution; offensive or heavy lochia or tachycardia. Women with two or more signs or symptoms require immediate referral for further evaluation (emergency action).

- If the pyrexia is not associated with other symptoms, gently palpate the abdomen; is there uterine pain during palpation? Are lochia heavy and/or offensive, have any large blood clots been passed? If infection is suspected, take HVS and dipstix analysis of urine and refer for further evaluation (urgent action).
- Even if there are no findings to indicate the presence of infection, the decision to refer must be at the healthcare professional's discretion.

## Abdominal tenderness

- Obtain history of onset and ask about condition of lochia. Gently palpate abdomen to establish the site of pain and assess involution. Is there any lower abdominal pain or generalised tenderness? Is the uterus positioned centrally or deviated, bulky or well contracted (findings could relate to number of postpartum days)? If subinvolution is suspected, take HVS and dipstix analysis of urine and refer (urgent action).

## Severe, life-threatening haemorrhage

If a woman is experiencing a severe haemorrhage at home the aim of immediate care must be to achieve prompt arrest of bleeding before the situation becomes critical.

- Massaging the uterus will aid expulsion of any clots and cause it to contract.
- Emergency medical aid must be summoned immediately (ambulance with paramedic support).
- If a woman is breastfeeding, put the baby to the breast.
- If there is time, empty the bladder with an indwelling catheter. Administer ergometrine 0.5 mg IM or IV if trained to do so (unless contraindicated, for example if woman has cardiovascular condition). If trained to do so, commence IV infusion.
- The obstetric unit should be informed of the need for admission.
- Information and reassurance should be given to the woman and her partner.
- Record all action taken.

# SUMMARY GUIDELINE

## Endometritis and abnormal blood loss

### Initial assessment – All women

- Obtain 'baseline' recording of involution
- Assess blood loss
- Note problems with delivery or third stage from delivery details

**Emergency action is required if:**

- Secondary PPH
- Tender and/or bulky uterus
- Pyrexia (temperature $>37.8°C$)
- Offensive lochia

Table 1.1    Summary of midwifery care for endometritis and abnormal bleeding

| Midwifery care | Abnormal bleeding | Offensive lochia |
|---|---|---|
| Establish | • Length of time heavier loss experienced | • Lochia are offensive |
| Exclude | • Associations with other factors, e.g. breastfeeding, rising up from lying or sitting | • Associations with other factors, e.g. infected perineal wound<br>• Poor personal hygiene |
| Ask the woman | • To describe amount of loss in inches or centimetres of spread on pad<br>• Is colour of loss different from previously?<br>• Is the loss offensive now, or has it been? | • Is colour of loss different from previously? |
| Describe and record | • Look at current pad<br>• Identify absorption level of pad used<br>• Describe the size of any clots passed, examine for placental tissues or membranes | |

**Record temperature and palpate uterus**

| ACTION | If normal: | If abnormal—raised temperature and/or pulse or uterine tenderness: |
|---|---|---|
| | • Reassure<br>• Monitor | • HVS<br>• MSU<br>• Refer to GP<br>• Advise mother about action taken and to contact midwife if symptoms become more severe |

## General advice

- Change maternity pads regularly, each time toilet visited if pads are stained, and at least four times a day for the first few days
- Blood loss may be heavy for the first few days, but it will gradually become less. It should have a non-offensive smell
- The healthcare professional should be contacted if the loss becomes:
  - heavier
  - bright red *after* the first week of delivery
  - offensive
- Analgesia should be taken if experiencing 'after pains' when breastfeeding

## References

Abbott H, Bick D, MacArthur C 1997 Health after birth. In: Henderson C, Jones K (eds) Essential midwifery. Mosby, London

AbouZahr C, Wardlaw T 2004 Maternal mortality in 2000: estimates developed by WHO, UNICEF and UNFPA. Available online at: www.who.int/reproductive-health/publications/maternal_mortality_2000/maternal_mortality_2000.pdf

Alexander J, Garcia J, Marchant S 1997 The BLiPP Study. A joint collaboration between the University of Portsmouth and the National Perinatal Epidemiology Unit, Oxford. Final Report to South & West NHS Executive Research and Development Committee. Institute of Health and Community Studies, Bournemouth

Alexander J, Thomas P, Sanghera J 2001 Treatments for secondary postpartum haemorrhage. Cochrane Database of Systematic Reviews, Issue 1. Update Software, Oxford

American College of Obstetricians and Gynecologists 1990 Technical bulletin. Diagnosis and management of postpartum haemorrhage. Int J Gynecol Obstet 36: 159-163

Bergstrom S, Libombo A 1992 Puerperal measurement of the symphysis–fundus distance. Gynecol Obstet Invest 34(2): 76-78

Bolling K, Grant C, Hamlyn B et al 2007 Infant feeding survey 2005. BMRB Social Research, London

Calhoun BC, Brost B 1995 Emergency management of sudden puerperal fever. Obstet Gynecol Clin North Am 22(2): 357-367

Carlan SJ, Scott WT, Pollack R, Harris K 1997 Appearance of the uterus by ultrasound immediately after placental delivery with pathologic correlation. J Clin Ultrasound 25(6): 301-308

Central Midwives Board 1962 Handbook incorporating the rules of the Central Midwives Board, 25th edn. William Clowes and Sons, London

Chaim W, Basiri A, Bar-David J et al 2000 Prevalence and clinical significance of postpartum endometritis and wound infection. Infect Dis Obstet Gynecol 8(2): 72-82

Cluett ER, Alexander J, Pickering RM 1995 Is measuring the symphysis fundal distance worthwhile? Midwifery 11(4): 174-183

Cluett ER, Alexander J, Pickering RM 1997 What is the normal pattern of uterine involution? An investigation of postpartum uterine involution measured by the distance between the symphysis pubis and the uterine fundus using a tape measure. Midwifery 13: 9-16

Ely JW, Dawson JD, Townsend AS et al 1996 Benign fever following vaginal delivery. J Fam Pract 43(2): 146-151

French LM, Smaill FM 2004 Antibiotic regimens for endometritis after delivery. Cochrane Database of Systematic Reviews, Issue 4

Fung ESM, Sin SY, Tang L 1996 Secondary postpartum haemorrhage: curettage or not? J Obstet Gynaecol 16(6): 514-517

Glazener CMA, Abdalla M, Stroud P et al 1995 Postnatal maternal morbidity: extent, causes, prevention and treatment. Br J Obstet Gynaecol 102(4): 282-287

Hertzberg B, Bowie J 1991 Ultrasound of the postpartum uterus. J Ultrasound Med 10: 451-456

Howie PW 1986 The puerperium and its complications. In: Whitfield CR (ed) Dewhirst's textbook of obstetrics and gynaecology for postgraduates. Blackwell Scientific Publications, Oxford.

Khan KS, Wojdyla D, Say L et al 2006 WHO analysis of causes of maternal deaths: a systematic review. Lancet 367: 1066-1074

Khong TY, Khong TK 1993 Delayed postpartum haemorrhage: a morphologic study of causes and their relation to other pregnancy disorders. Obstet Gynecol 82(1): 17-22

Khong TY, De Wolf F, Robertson WB et al 1986 Inadequate vascular response to placentation in pregnancies complicated by pre-eclampsia and by small-for-gestational age infants. Br J Obstet Gynaecol 93: 1049-1059

Lee CY, Madrazo B, Drukker BH 1981 Ultrasonic evaluation of the postpartum uterus in the management of postpartum bleeding. Obstet Gynecol 58(2): 227-232

Lewis G, Drife J 2004 Why mothers die 2000–2002. Report on confidential enquiries into maternal deaths in the United Kingdom. Royal College of Obstetricians and Gynaecologists, London

MacArthur C, Lewis M, Knox EG 1991 Health after childbirth. HMSO, London

Marchant S, Alexander J 1996 Midwives' assessment of postnatal uterine involution – is it of value? International Congress of Midwives, Conference Proceedings. 24th Triennial Conference, Oslo

Marchant S, Alexander J, Garcia J 1996 Postnatal observations (letter). Midwives 109(1302): 204

Marchant S, Alexander J, Garcia J et al 1999 A survey of women's experiences of vaginal loss from 24 hours to three months of childbirth (the BliPP study). Midwifery 15: 72-81

Marchant S, Alexander J, Garcia J 2002 Postnatal vaginal bleeding problems and general practice. Midwifery 18: 21-24

Montgomery E, Alexander J 1994 Assessing postnatal uterine involution: a review and a challenge. Midwifery 10: 73-76

National Institute for Health and Clinical Excellence (NICE) 2006 Postnatal care: routine postnatal care of women and their babies. Nice Clinical Guideline 37.

Oppenheimer LW, Sherriff EA, Goodman JDS et al 1986 The duration of lochia. Br J Obstet Gynaecol 93: 754-757

Parrott T, Evans AJ, Lowes A et al 1989 Infection following caesarean section. J Hosp Infect 13: 349-354

Pastorek JG, Sanders CV 1991 Antibiotic therapy for postcaesarean endomyometritis. Rev Infect Dis 13 (suppl 9): S752-S757

Pijnenborg R, Anthony J, Davey DA et al 1991 Placental bed spiral arteries in the hypertensive disorders of pregnancy. Br J Obstet Gynaecol 98: 655-658

Robertson PA, Huang LJ, Croughan-Minihane MS et al 1998 Is there an association between water baths during labor and the development of chorioamnionitis or endometritis? Am J Obstet Gynecol 178(6): 1215-1221

Rome RM 1975 Secondary postpartum haemorrhage. J Obstet Gynaecol 82: 289-292

Royal College of Midwives (RCM) 2002 Successful breastfeeding, 3rd edn. Churchill Livingstone, Edinburgh

Schuurmans N, MacKinnon C, Lane C et al 2000 SOCG clinical practice guidelines. Prevention and management of postpartum haemorrhage. J Human Lactation 15: 35-39

Smaill F, Hofmeyr GJ 2000 Antibiotic prophylaxis for caesarean section. Cochrane Library of Systematic Reviews, Issue 3

Tekay A, Joupila P 1993 A longitudinal doppler ultrasonographic assessment of the alterations in peripheral vascular resistance of the uterine arteries and ultrasonographic findings of the involuting uterus during the puerperium. Am J Obstet Gynecol 168: 190-198

Visness CM, Kennedy KI, Ramos R 1997 The duration and character of postpartum bleeding among breast-feeding women. Obstet Gynecol 89(2): 159-163

World Health Organization 2003 Vaginal bleeding after childbirth. In: Managing complications in pregnancy and childbirth: a guide for midwives and doctors. World Health Organization, Geneva

World Health Organization 2006 Pregnancy, childbirth, postpartum and newborn care: a guide for essential practice. World Health Organization, Geneva

Yokoe DS, Christiansen CI, Johnson R et al 2001 Epidemiology of and surveillance for postpartum infections. Emerg Infect Dis 7: 1-5

## Chapter 2

# Perineal pain and dyspareunia

## INTRODUCTION

The majority of women who have a vaginal delivery will experience some degree of perineal pain, which is one of the most commonly reported symptoms in the immediate postnatal period (Sleep 1995). Dyspareunia or painful sexual intercourse, although a different symptom, can be related to perineal pain. Several of the relevant studies, especially those with information on risk factors, have investigated both of these symptoms. If each symptom were to be reviewed and described separately in this guideline, there would be substantial repetition. Some parts of the guideline therefore describe perineal pain and dyspareunia in separate sections and others describe them together. In addition to dyspareunia, there are some recent data on other sexual health problems after childbirth and on the timing of the resumption of sexual intercourse, which are also described in this guideline.

## Definitions

- **Perineal pain** is defined as any pain occurring in the perineal body, an area of muscular and fibrous tissue which extends from the symphysis pubis to the coccyx.
- **Dyspareunia** refers to pain or discomfort occurring during sexual intercourse, including pain on penetration. Dyspareunia is sometimes categorised as superficial or deep.

## Frequency of occurrence: perineal pain

Information on the prevalence of perineal pain is available from several observational studies based on representative samples and with adequate response rates. A number of trials which have investigated various forms of perineal management including perineal pain as an outcome measure have also provided some data, although it is important to keep in mind that whilst trials provide best evidence on causality, if trial inclusion is restricted to particular types of delivery, this limits the generalisability of the prevalence estimates.

Pain has been assessed using a number of tools developed for use in the general population, including visual analogue scales and visual assessment tools. In one randomised controlled trial (RCT) (Kettle et al 2002), pain measures at 10 days after the birth included levels of pain experienced by women on activity, including when passing urine and opening their bowels. Other indicators of pain severity have included total dosage of analgesia used, weight of total amount of topically applied anaesthesia and/or frequency of treatments. The timing of assessment of perineal pain often differs between studies and there is limited information on the long-term effects of pain.

In a prospective observational study in Scotland, among a representative sample of all deliveries over a defined period, 42% of 1249 women reported a painful perineum when questioned in hospital (Glazener et al 1995). In the West Berkshire Perineal Management Trial (see later), 23% of almost 900 women (inclusion restricted to those expected to have a spontaneous vaginal delivery (SVD)) reported perineal pain at 10 days postpartum (Sleep et al 1984). Among over 5000 spontaneous vaginal births in the 'hands on or poised' trial (HOOP), which compared alternative methods of conducting the second stage of labour, 33% of women in the trial as a whole reported perineal pain in the previous 24 hours, when asked at 10 days postpartum (McCandlish et al 1998). A prospective cohort study from Canada, which examined differences in perineal pain relative to the type of trauma sustained among 444 women who had a vaginal birth, found that overall 92% reported pain on the first day after the birth and 61% reported pain on day 7 (Macarthur & Macarthur 2004).

Perineal pain is clearly very common in the early puerperium, but for some women it can also be more persistent and various studies have shown that at least 8–10% of women experience this well past the 6–8-week postnatal discharge from maternity care. In the trial by Sleep et al (1984), when followed up at 3 months, 8% of the women reported perineal pain at that time. In the study by Glazener et al (1995), when questioned again at 8 weeks, 22% of the sample reported experiencing a painful perineum between then and the first week, and when questioned at 12–18 months, 9.8% had experienced perineal pain at some time between 8 weeks and 12–18 months. Brown & Lumley (1998) contacted 1336 women at 6–7 months postpartum in a cross-sectional study of all deliveries occurring over 2 weeks within a region in Australia, and found that for 21% a painful perineum had been a problem at some time since the birth. The proportion who still had this at 6–7 months was not given. Macarthur & Macarthur (2004) reported that 7% of women in their study population had perineal pain when questioned about this at 6 weeks after the birth.

## Frequency of occurrence: dyspareunia

Like perineal pain, there is some information on the prevalence of dyspareunia from observational studies and from the trials of perineal management, although again it must be remembered that data on this from samples restricted to particular delivery-types or parity groups will limit the generalisability of the estimates obtained.

Brown & Lumley (1998), in the Australian study described earlier, found that 26% of the women questioned at 6–7 months postpartum had experienced 'a sexual problem' at some time since the birth, although further specification of the problem was not given nor what proportion still had it. Glazener (1997) found that at 8 weeks postpartum, 25% of the sample had not attempted intercourse. The remaining 75% had attempted intercourse although for 5% it had been unsuccessful. Questions on problems with intercourse were included, showing that between 1 and 8 weeks, 28% of women had found intercourse to be sore or difficult; between 2–18 months this was reported by 20%. Lack of interest in sex was reported by 9% of women at 8 weeks, rising to 21% between 2–18 months.

A cross-sectional study of all primiparous women delivering in one maternity unit in London was conducted to enquire about a range of sexual health problems (Barrett et al 2000). Postal questionnaires were sent at 6 months postpartum to 796 primiparae asking about sexual problems since the birth and prior to pregnancy; 484 (61%) replied. By 6 weeks (as recalled), 32% of women had resumed intercourse, 62% had done so by 8 weeks and 81% by 3 months. Dyspareunia, which was specified as including painful penetration and/or pain during intercourse or orgasm, was experienced by 62% of women at some time in the first 3 months after birth and 31% still had this at 6 months. Loss of sexual desire was reported by 53% of women in the first 3 months, and by 37% at 6 months. Other problems still experienced at 6 months were vaginal tightness (20%), vaginal looseness or lack of muscle tone (12%) and lack of vaginal lubrication (26%). Enquiry was also made about the same set of sexual problems in relation to the year before pregnancy and, although subject to greater recall bias, all problems were found to have increased significantly in the first 3 months after delivery. Although all problems had declined by 6 months postpartum, they were still substantially greater than pre-pregnancy levels. The response rate in this survey was 61%, which is good given the sensitive nature of the subject, but gives less confidence in relation to prevalence estimates. Even if all of the non-responders were problem free, however, the findings still provide clear evidence that sexual problems are common as well as persistent following childbirth.

Sleep et al (1984), in their trial, found that by 3 months postpartum 90% of women reported having resumed sexual intercourse. Just over half of these had experienced dyspareunia at some time since the birth and almost 20% still had it at 3 months. Klein et al (1994), in a similar trial (see later), found that 64% of the sample had resumed intercourse by 6 weeks and 96% by 3 months. On first intercourse, almost 80% of the women reported some pain, although in most cases this was only mild or discomforting.

## Risk factors: perineal pain and dyspareunia

The main risk factors for perineal pain and dyspareunia that have been identified in studies relate to mode of delivery, perineal trauma and primiparity. These factors are all clearly highly interrelated so appropriate multivariate analyses need to be undertaken in order to report on the independent effects of each. Methods of managing perineal trauma, such as the use of different suture methods and materials, have also been investigated with respect to subsequent perineal pain and dyspareunia and are described in this section on risk factors.

### *Mode of delivery*

Mode of delivery is associated with substantial variation in perineal pain (short and long term) with much higher rates occurring after instrumental compared with spontaneous vaginal deliveries and the lowest rates occurring after caesarean sections. There is a similar pattern for reporting of dyspareunia but differences are generally less marked. There has been increasing debate on the benefits and risks of planned caesarean section compared with vaginal birth, with one of the purported reasons for offering women a choice over mode of birth being impact of vaginal birth on perineal trauma and sexual health.

In the study by Glazener et al (1995) described earlier, differences in perineal pain according to delivery mode were clearly documented, occurring whilst still in hospital, between then and 8 weeks, and between 2 and 18 months. The respective prevalences whilst in hospital were 84% after instrumental delivery, 42% after an SVD and 5% after caesarean section; 59%, 19% and 4% between then and 8 weeks; and 30%, 7% and 2% between 2 and 18 months. Data on dyspareunia were also reported for this sample (see earlier), but not separately according to mode of delivery (Glazener 1997).

Johanson et al (1993) obtained data on a number of morbidity indicators from 313 women who were part of an RCT of forceps versus vacuum extraction deliveries, and from 100 consecutive unselected SVD deliveries. A significant difference in perineal discomfort at 24–48 hours was found, which occurred in 45% of the instrumental delivery group and 28% of the SVD group (odds ratio (OR) 2.1, 95% confidence interval (CI) 1.2–3.4). At 15–24 months postpartum, 28% compared with 19% respectively reported a painful perineum (mostly occurring only sometimes), but this difference was not statistically significant. Pain on intercourse (mostly occurring only sometimes) at 15–24 months, however, was significantly more common in the instrumental group, reported by 37%, compared with 21% of the normal deliveries (OR 2.0, 95% CI 1.03–3.80).

Brown & Lumley (1998), in their population-based sample in Australia, found that perineal pain, reported as a problem some time between the birth and 6–7 months postpartum, occurred in 20% of women after SVD, 54% after instrumental birth, 2% after emergency caesarean section and none after elective section (OR for instrumental relative to SVD 4.69, 95% CI 3.2–6.8). Sexual problems, not further specified, differed only for instrumental deliveries, being reported by 24%, 39%, 29% and 27% respectively after the four types of delivery (OR for instrumental relative to SVD 2.06, 95% CI 1.4–3.0). These differences in perineal pain and sexual problems between instrumental compared with spontaneous vaginal births were adjusted to take account of infant birthweight, length of labour and degree of perineal trauma, and remained statistically significant.

Signorello and colleagues (2001), in a study from Boston, Massachusetts which recruited primiparous women, reported an OR of 2.5 (95% CI 1.3–4.8) of dyspareunia at 6 months after giving birth following assisted vaginal delivery compared with spontaneous vaginal delivery. This was after adjusting data for maternal age, method of infant feeding, prior experience of dyspareunia, duration of the second stage of labour, extent of perineal trauma and infant birthweight.

A German study evaluated the impact of mode of delivery on sexual health among primiparous women with responses from 655 of 1613 (41%) women contacted from 6 months to 2.5 years after the birth (Buhling et al 2006). The researchers found that 47% of women had resumed intercourse within 8 weeks of birth, and although 69% (436/633) reported some pain on resumption, the degree of pain differed significantly by mode of delivery. Women who had an operative vaginal delivery had a higher prevalence of pain compared with women who had a caesarean section or spontaneous vaginal birth without perineal injury (p<0.007). The potential for response bias and failure to take account of potential confounding factors in the analysis means findings should be interpreted with caution.

Barrett et al (2000), in their study of sexual problems among primiparae, found that dyspareunia occurring some time during the first 3 months postpartum was reported by 62% of women after an SVD, 78% after forceps/ventouse delivery, 41% after a section with labour and 47% after a section without labour. After adjustment for possible confounders, the difference for forceps/ventouse deliveries relative to SVD remained significant (OR 2.41, 95% CI 1.24–4.69), but the differences for both types of caesarean section did not. Dyspareunia at 6 months postpartum was reported by 30% of women after SVD, 37% after forceps/ventouse and 28% and 21% respectively after section with and without labour, but none of these differences was statistically significant. Continued breastfeeding up to 6 months was one of the two factors in this study found to be significantly associated with dyspareunia at 6 months. The other was a previous history of dyspareunia prior to pregnancy and both factors remained significant after logistic adjustment. Among the women still breastfeeding, 40% reported dyspareunia compared with 25% of those not breastfeeding (OR 2.25, 95% CI 1.42–3.57). The researchers suggest that hormonal profile, loss of libido and vaginal dryness could contribute towards the symptom excess in breastfeeding mothers.

Glazener (1997) found that women who were still breastfeeding at 8 weeks were significantly more likely to report a lack of interest in intercourse than those who were bottle feeding. Tiredness was also more common among the breastfeeding mothers, but even after taking account of this, the relationship with lack of interest in sex remained.

A recent small study compared perineal morbidity and sexual function following vaginal delivery or elective caesarean section (Griffiths et al 2006). Two hundred and eight women were contacted 2 years after delivery of their first baby to record the prevalence of a number of subjective physical and psychological health problems, including sexual satisfaction. Exclusion criteria included women who had had a subsequent pregnancy. Replies were received from 109 women (52%). The proportions of women reporting all symptoms of interest within the 2-year period, including dyspareunia, were higher among women who had given birth vaginally. Dyspareunia was reported by 33% of women in the spontaneous vaginal delivery group, 36% in the ventouse group and 52% in the forceps group, with no cases reported among the elective caesarean section group. Women who had dyspareunia were asked about the severity of this (information on how questions were asked was not provided), which showed that severity was highest among women who had a forceps delivery. Findings should be interpreted with caution due to the low response rate, small numbers, potential for recall bias in relation to when symptoms were first experienced and lack of analysis to enable independent risk factors to be identified.

*Perineal trauma*

Perineal trauma is generally considered to be more likely to result in perineal pain and dyspareunia than if the perineum is intact, but there has been considerable debate on the benefits and adverse effects of episiotomy compared with spontaneous laceration (Sleep 1995). Several trials have examined this issue. The West Berkshire Perineal Management Trial (Sleep et al 1984), referred to earlier, of a restricted versus a liberal episiotomy policy, was the first to provide good evidence on the effects of episiotomy use among women who, towards the end of second-stage labour, were expected to have a spontaneous vaginal delivery. For women allocated to the restrictive group, the midwife was asked to avoid episiotomy and only perform an incision if fetal indications (bradycardia, tachycardia, meconium-stained liquor) warranted this (n = 498). In the liberal group the midwife was asked to try to prevent a perineal tear (n = 502), the intention being that she should use episiotomy more liberally to do this. The different policies did result in more tears and more intact perinea in the restrictive group, but no differences were found in perineal pain at 10 days or 3 months, nor in dyspareunia at 3 months. These authors concluded that the findings provide little support for either the liberal use of episiotomy or for claims that its reduced use would decrease postpartum morbidity (Sleep et al 1984).

Klein et al (1994) carried out a similar trial in Canada, which again found that although significantly fewer episiotomies were performed in the restrictive policy group, there were no differences at 1 and 10 days postpartum in perineal pain, or in sexual problems (pain and sexual satisfaction) at 3 months.

A Cochrane systematic review (Carroli et al 2000) including six RCTs comparing policies of the restrictive use of episiotomy versus routine/liberal use confirmed that there were no differences in perineal pain or dyspareunia according to episiotomy policy, although other differences (reduced risk of posterior perineal trauma, less suturing and fewer healing complications) led the reviewers to conclude that a restrictive episiotomy policy was beneficial and should be recommended.

Since these trials were comparing perineal management policies, some women in the restricted episiotomy group still had an episiotomy, and vice versa. In the study by Klein et al (1994), it was felt that this justified undertaking further subgroup analyses and all women in the trial were recategorised (irrespective of trial group allocation) according to the type of perineal trauma (intact, laceration, episiotomy, third/fourth-degree tears). Perineal pain between days 1–10 and at 3 months was found to be least in the intact group and greatest in those with third/fourth-degree tears. Episiotomy and spontaneous tears were intermediate and differed from each other for early perineal pain and for later pain classed as occurring most or all of the time, both a little more common after episiotomy. Dyspareunia on first resumption of intercourse followed a similar pattern of relationship with trauma. The type of episiotomy in this trial was midline, which is rarely practised in the UK, and almost all women in the trial had spontaneous vaginal deliveries.

In a subsequent analysis of data from the study by Glazener (1997) to determine the independent predictors of pain or difficulty with intercourse at 2 months postpartum, logistic regression was undertaken and episiotomy was found to be an independent predictor of this (Glazener 1998).

The prospective cohort study from Canada (Macarthur & Macarthur 2004) which collected data on perineal pain outcomes from 447 women of all parities who had given birth vaginally, at 1 day, 7 days and 6 weeks after the birth, included 84 women who had an intact perineum, 220 who had a first- or second-degree tear, 97 women who had an episiotomy (including women who had either a midline or mediolateral episiotomy) and 46 who had a third- or fourth-degree tear. The primary study outcome was the incidence of perineal pain on the day of interview, with secondary outcomes including pain score measurements and impact of pain on daily activities. There were high response rates at each stage of the study (95% or above). Multivariable regression analysis was undertaken to calculate adjusted relative risks, after taking account of differences between the groups on potential confounding variables. Acute postpartum perineal pain was common among all women but pain severity was more frequent and more severe for women who had more extensive perineal trauma. On day 1, the three groups of women who had sustained trauma were 30% more likely to report pain, and on day 7 the adjusted RR of perineal pain in the trauma groups compared with the intact group ranged from 1.5 (first- or second-degree tear) to 2.1 (third- or fourth-degree tear).

## Parity

Perineal pain and dyspareunia have both been documented as more common after first compared with subsequent births (Barrett et al 1998, Glazener et al 1995). However, the extent to which this is influenced by the greater proportion of instrumental deliveries and perineal trauma that occur among first births is difficult to assess. The parity association found by Glazener et al (1995) for painful perineum was based on univariate analysis, not taking other factors into account. For pain or difficulty with intercourse at 2 months postpartum, multivariate analysis was undertaken to take account of possible interrelated factors and showed that primiparity remained associated with the symptoms, although forceps delivery did not. In the perineal management trial by Sleep et al (1984), data were presented separately for first and later births showing that mild and moderate perineal pain at 10 days were reported by almost twice as many primiparae as multiparae. This study was of anticipated spontaneous vaginal births so should not be confounded by any parity-related instrumental delivery effect, but in both trial arms the primiparae had more perineal trauma (episiotomy or laceration) than the multiparae. Klein et al (1994), in their similar study, stated that primiparae experienced more perineal pain and sexual problems than multiparae, but presented no data to show this.

## Suture materials and methods

The effects of suture materials and methods on subsequent perineal pain and dyspareunia have been examined in a number of systematic reviews, some of which have had clear findings relevant to practice.

A Cochrane systematic review, including eight RCTs, compared synthetic suture materials with catgut (Kettle & Johanson 1999). Catgut is manufactured from collagen from mammals and has been a commonly used suture material, whilst synthetic suture materials, polyglycolic acid (Dexon) and polyglactin (Vicryl), are more recent. All the trials in the review were consistent in showing lower rates of short-term (3 days) perineal pain in the synthetic suture groups (OR 0.62, 95% CI 0.54–0.71). Two of the trials examined perineal pain and three examined dyspareunia at 3 months, with no differences found in either of these longer term outcomes according to type of suture material. Other outcomes, the need for analgesia and suture dehiscence, were reduced in the groups sutured with synthetic material, but two trials that included as secondary outcomes the removal of suture material at 10 days and 3 months found this was undertaken more often in the synthetic materials group. The reviewers concluded that the use of absorbable synthetic suture material (polyglycolic acid and polyglactin sutures) appears to decrease short-term perineal pain. The length of time taken for synthetic material to be absorbed, however, is of concern (Kettle & Johanson 1999).

The effects of continuous subcuticular versus interrupted transcutaneous sutures for closure of perineal skin on long- and short-term perineal pain and dyspareunia, and a number of other outcomes, were examined in a recently updated Cochrane systematic review (Kettle et al 2007). Seven trials, which provided data on 3822 women, were included. Meta-analysis showed that continuous suture techniques (all layers or perineal skin only) were associated with less pain for up to 10 days postpartum (relative risk (RR) 0.70, 95% CI 0.64–0.76) when compared with interrupted sutures for perineal closure. Subgroup analysis showed greater reduction in pain when continuous suturing techniques were used for all layers (RR 0.65, 95% CI 0.60–0.71). There was an overall reduction in analgesia use associated with the continuous subcutaneous technique compared with interrupted sutures for repair of perineal skin (RR 0.70, 95% CI 0.58 0.84). There was some evidence of reduction in dyspareunia up to 3 months after the birth experienced by women in the groups who had continuous suturing for all layers of their perineal trauma (RR 0.83, 95% CI 0.70–0.98). There was also a reduction in suture removal in the continuous suturing groups versus interrupted (RR 0.54, 95% CI 0.45–0.65) but no significant differences in the need for resuturing of wounds or long-term pain.

A stratified RCT (Ipswich Childbirth Study – included in the systematic review described above of type of suture material), used a 2 × 2 factorial design and also compared the effects of the standard three-stage suturing with a two-stage method, in which the perineal skin was left unsutured (Gordon et al 1998). The trial was carried out in a single centre and involved 1780 women of all parities who sustained episiotomy or first- or second-degree tears following spontaneous or instrumental vaginal deliveries. Women were assessed by questionnaire at 24–48 hours, 10 days and 3 months postpartum. No differences were found in perineal pain at 24–48 hours or 10 days between the two- and three-stage repair groups, but at 3 months fewer women in the two-stage group reported perineal pain and more had resumed pain-free intercourse. Among women who had resumed intercourse, reduced rates of dyspareunia in the two-stage group just reached statistical significance (RR 0.80, 95% CI 0.65–0.99).

In a large RCT undertaken at a hospital in North Staffordshire, which also used a 2 × 2 factorial design (included in the above review of suturing methods, but not included in the review of suture materials), Kettle et al (2002) randomised 1542 women who had a spontaneous vaginal delivery with a second-degree tear or episiotomy to either a continuous (n = 771) or inter-rupted (n = 771) suturing method, and to be sutured using either a rapidly absorbed polyglactin 910 suture material (n = 772) or standard polyglactin 910 (n = 770). Primary outcomes were pain at 10 days after giving birth, and superficial dyspareunia at 3 months. There was significantly less peri-neal pain amongst women who had a continuous technique at 10 days (OR 0.47, 95% CI 0.38–0.58), the researchers postulating that the pain reduc-tion may be a consequence of the transfer of tension along the whole of the single suture and avoidance of nerve endings as skin sutures are inserted into subcutaneous tissue. There were no differences in the reporting of pain according to the type of suture material used. At 3 months there were no dif-ferences in the reporting of superficial dyspareunia between women whose trauma had been sutured using the continuous or interrupted methods (OR 0.84, 95% CI 0.72–1.33) or among the rapidly absorbed suture material or standard suture material groups (OR 1.13, 95% CI 0.84–1.54). Suture mate-rial was less likely to have been removed among women in the rapidly absorbed material group and in the continuous suture method group. The researchers concluded that use of the continuous repair methods could pre-vent one in six women from experiencing perineal pain at 10 days after birth, and use of the rapidly absorbed polyglactin 910 material could obviate the need for suture removal within the first 3 months for one in 10 women sutured.

Another aspect of perineal management, this time in relation to the benefit of techniques to support the perineum during the expulsive phase of a vagi-nal birth with cephalic presentation, was evaluated in one RCT. Perineal pain at 10 days as the main outcome measure and pain and dyspareunia at 3 months were included as secondary outcomes (McCandlish et al 1998). This was the HOOP trial ('hands on or poised'), in which 5471 women were randomised to being delivered with the 'hands on' (the midwife put pres-sure on the baby's head and 'guarded' the perineum; n = 2731) or the 'hands poised' method (the midwife kept her hands poised, not touching the baby's head or the perineum, allowing spontaneous delivery of the shoulders; n = 2740). At 10 days postpartum significantly more women in the 'hands poised' group (34.1%) reported perineal pain in the previous 24 hours com-pared with the 'hands on' group (31.1%), although this difference was great-est in the 'mild' pain category. There was no difference in perineal pain or in dyspareunia at 3 months. Other outcomes, including urinary problems, bowel problems and postnatal depression, did not vary between groups but episiotomy rates were significantly higher in the 'hands on' group, and manual removal of the placenta significantly lower.

Until recently, it was commonly accepted that all perineal trauma should be sutured to restore the integrity and function of perineal tissue (McCandl-ish 2001). One anecdotal consequence of concerns relating to high levels of perineal morbidity has been the growing number of clinicians and women who have questioned the need to suture all second-degree tears, despite lim-ited evidence to support a change in practice. Two small RCTs compared suturing versus non-suturing of second-degree tears (Fleming et al 2003, Lundquist et al 2000). Lundquist et al (2000) randomised 80 primiparous women to be sutured or not sutured, collecting data on pain, discomfort and dyspareunia at 2–3 days, 8 days and 6 months after birth. Results showed that 'small' unsutured tears healed as well as sutured ones but the definition and measurement of healing were not clarified. Fleming and colleagues (2003) randomised 74 primiparous women who sustained a first- or second-degree tear to be sutured or not sutured. Perineal pain and wound healing were assessed at 1 and 10 days and 6 weeks postpartum. No significant differences were found in reported pain, but significantly more women in the sutured group had good wound approximation at 6 weeks (p<0.001), further analysis showing that suturing and a shorter labour increased the odds of wound approximation. The small sample limits the generalisability of the study findings.

In the largest observational study to date to have compared outcomes in relation to suturing or non-suturing of perineal trauma in routine practice, 282 women were followed from birth to 12 months, to capture data on a range of outcomes to ascertain if there were differences in physical or psychological health and well-being (Metcalfe et al 2006). Primiparous and multiparous women who had a spontaneous vaginal delivery and sustained a second-degree tear were asked about health outcomes at 24 hours, 10 days, 12 weeks and 12 months after giving birth. One hundred and ninety six (70%) women had their trauma sutured and 86 (30%) had trauma unsutured, the decision to suture or not being based on the midwife's clinical judgement and practice. There were no significant differences in perineal pain outcomes, use of analgesia or other types of pain relief or perineal wound infection at any of the four time points by suture or non-suture group. Women in the sutured group resumed intercourse earlier (mean 40.72 days, 95% CI 39.27–42.16) than the unsutured group (mean 44.02 days, 95% CI 41.86–46.18) but this difference was not significant. The researchers concluded that results should be interpreted with caution, given the low recruitment rate (only around 20% of women eligible were recruited). Nevertheless, findings suggested that all second-degree tears should continue to be sutured until evidence from large RCTs is available and work to ascertain women's views of perineal management has been undertaken.

## Management: perineal pain

### Topically applied anaesthetics

The effectiveness of topically applied anaesthetics for relief of perineal pain in hospital and following postnatal discharge was examined in a Cochrane systematic review (Hedayati et al 2005). Eight trials were included, presenting data on 976 women. Five trials measured pain experienced up to 24 hours after giving birth, although each trial used a different method to assess pain levels. All five trials showed no difference in pain relief when the topical anaesthetic was compared with placebo, based on short-term pain relief. Two trials looked at use of additional analgesia for perineal pain relief, one trial finding that less additional analgesia was required with use of Epifoam in comparison with placebo (RR 0.58, 95% CI 0.40–0.84, one trial with 97 women). Use of lignocaine/lidocaine showed no difference with regard to the requirement for additional analgesia. Evidence to support use of topical applications is not robust and further work is required.

## Oral analgesia

In a survey by Sleep & Grant (1988a) oral analgesia (usually paracetamol) was the first-line treatment for mild perineal pain in 78% of the 50 maternity units investigated. Sleep (1995), in a review of postnatal perineal care, noted that several factors need to be considered when deciding on the most appropriate oral preparation, including an assessment of the severity of the pain, the potential for the analgesia to be secreted into breast milk and possible side-effects, such as constipation or nausea.

Among the women who responded to a NCT survey of women's experiences and midwifery practices in relation to perineal care (Greenshields & Hulme 1993), of those who had used oral analgesia to relieve perineal pain, the majority considered paracetamol to be the most effective. Other oral analgesia taken by women in this survey included aspirin, ibuprofen, codeine and coproxamol. Effectiveness of simple oral analgesia is considered in more detail under pain relief following caesarean section (p. 50).

## Rectal analgesia

A Cochrane review of rectal analgesia for pain from perineal trauma following childbirth (Hedayati et al 2003) included data on 249 women from three trials. Two trials, both from the UK, compared diclofenac suppositories with placebo, while the third trial (from Saudi Arabia) compared indometacin with placebo. Only the two trials from the UK provided data appropriate for use in a meta-analysis. Women were less likely to experience pain at or close to 24 hours after giving birth if they had received non-steroidal anti-inflammatory drug (NSAID) suppositories compared with placebo. In the two UK trials, women who had received the NSAID suppositories were also less likely to require additional analgesia in the first 24 hours after giving birth and, based on data from one UK trial, this effect was still evident at 48 hours postbirth. There was no information on pain experienced more than 72 hours after the birth, impact on other activities, resumption of intercourse or mother–infant relationship.

There is clearly some benefit from the use of diclofenac rectal suppositories for perineal pain relief but larger studies are required to confirm these findings, to assess longer term effects, maternal satisfaction, effectiveness for women with trauma following instrumental delivery and as a therapeutic measure for those already experiencing perineal pain.

## Bathing

One small trial compared the effects on perineal pain of sitting in either warm or cold baths (Ramler & Roberts 1986). This found that whilst cold baths were significantly more effective in relieving perineal pain, especially straight after delivery, the effect was limited to the first half hour of treatment and few women would want to sit in a cold bath – 119 of 159 women approached refused to take part in the trial.

A remedy traditionally considered to relieve perineal pain and enhance wound healing has been the addition of salt to bath water. A three-arm RCT examined the effectiveness of adding salt, a 25 ml sachet of 'Savlon' or nothing to the bath water each day for the first 10 days, among 1800 vaginal deliveries (Sleep & Grant 1988b). The prevalence of perineal pain and pattern of wound healing at 10 days were similar in all groups and at 3 months perineal pain, timing of resumption of intercourse or dyspareunia did not differ either. Using salt or 'Savlon' bath additives therefore cannot be recommended to reduce pain or dyspareunia or to enhance healing, but over 90% of women in each of the groups reported at 10 days that they had found bathing to be helpful in relieving their perineal discomfort.

## Alternative therapies

There is anecdotal evidence from women that some alternative remedies, such as arnica and lavender oil, provide relief of perineal pain (Greenshields & Hulme 1993). Dale & Cornwell (1994) conducted an RCT including 635 women, which compared adding pure lavender oil, synthetic lavender oil or an inert oil to bath water on each of the first 10 days postpartum. Daily discomfort scores were assessed using a visual analogue scale but no significant differences between the groups were found. Further trials are required to assess the safety and benefit of alternative remedies before they can be recommended as effective for the relief of perineal pain.

## Use of ice packs and cooling gel pads

Ice packs have been commonly used to reduce inflammation of acute soft tissue injury, and are reported to be the most commonly used form of local treatment of perineal pain (Greenshields & Hulme 1993). There does not appear to be a standard ice pack used in postnatal care, but numerous locally made applications (often prepared by staff on the postnatal ward) include the fingers of latex gloves and crushed ice 'sandwiched' between layers of gauze. There have been some concerns about side-effects of the use of ice on soft tissue, including vasoconstriction (Sleep 1990), although evidence to support this is not available. Another concern is that ice packs cannot be moulded to the shape of the perineum.

An RCT undertaken by Steen et al (2000) compared the effectiveness of a specifically developed cooling device (maternity gel pad) on reduction of perineal pain, compared with ice packs and Epifoam. One hundred and twenty women who had an instrumental delivery were recruited from a maternity unit in the north of England and randomised to one of three treatment groups: ice packs only (n = 38); Epifoam only (n = 42); and gel pads only (n = 40). Women could continue to use other forms of pain relief if they wished, including oral analgesia and bathing, and apply the treatments they were allocated to as required.

The main study outcomes included levels of oedema, bruising and self-assessed pain as measured using specifically developed scales at different time points during the postnatal period. These included a visual evaluating tool (Steen & Cooper 1997) used by midwife assessors blinded to treatment allocation to ascertain levels of perineal oedema and bruising at $\leq 4$ hours, 24 hours and 48 hours, and a 10-point VAS to capture data on self-assessed pain at $\leq 4$, 24 and 48 hours. Pain at 5 days after suturing was also collected using the VAS, which was recorded by community midwives. Women's opinions on the effectiveness of the treatment they received were rated using a 5-point scale of poor, fair, good, very good and excellent. The majority of women in each group had signs of perineal oedema within 4 hours of birth, with no treatment effect identified within the first 4 hours or at 24 hours. There was a significant difference in oedema at 48 hours, women in the gel pad treatment group having less oedema compared with either of the standard regimens. Women in the gel pad group who initially reported moderate or severe pain had significantly less pain at 48 hours. There was no difference in treatment effect across the groups at other initial levels of severity of oedema, bruising or pain at 24 and 48 hours or pain levels at 5 days. Women allocated to the maternity gel pad group were more likely to rate their treatment as effective. The researchers concluded that the gel pads were more effective at relieving pain compared with standard treatment regimens, and more highly rated by the women. As treatments were only administered on the postnatal ward, effectiveness in the community is difficult to predict but given the known duration of perineal pain as described earlier in this section, further work should be undertaken.

## Ultrasound

There is some evidence of the effectiveness of ultrasound in the treatment of soft tissue injuries from studies of general populations (Binder et al 1985), and ultrasound and pulsed electromagnetic therapy are now increasingly used as treatments to relieve acute perineal pain. Ultrasound is thought to reduce pain by resolution of the inflammation process and reduction of pressure from haematoma and oedema on pain sensitive structures (Hay-Smith 2000). In the survey of obstetric units described earlier (Sleep & Grant 1988a), 36% reported using ultrasound and 6% pulsed electromagnetic therapy.

Hay-Smith (2000), in a Cochrane systematic review of four trials of therapeutic ultrasound involving 659 women, reported that based on two placebo-controlled trials, women with acute perineal pain treated by active ultrasound were more likely to report improvement (OR 0.37, 95% CI 0.19–0.69). One trial of ultrasound compared with electromagnetic therapy found that those treated with ultrasound were less likely to have perineal pain at 10 days and 3 months (OR 0.43, 95% CI 0.22–0.84), although they were more likely to have bruising at 10 days (OR 1.64, 95% CI 1.04–2.60). One trial examined treatment for dyspareunia presenting at 6 weeks or later and found that this was more likely to be relieved after ultrasound than placebo but fewer women in the ultrasound group had attempted intercourse. The reviewer concluded that there is not enough good-quality evidence to adequately evaluate the effects of ultrasound in treating perineal pain and dyspareunia. However, in view of the potential benefit of ultrasound in general wound healing, the reviewer did suggest that further high-quality trials were warranted.

## Cushions and rings

Sometimes women are advised to ease perineal pain and discomfort by sitting on a rubber or sorbo ring, but there is little evidence of the effectiveness of these commonly used aides (Sleep 1995).

## Pelvic floor muscle exercises (PFME)

Sleep & Grant (1987) conducted a trial including 1800 women to assess the effects of intensive compared with routine pelvic floor exercises on various outcomes at 3 months postpartum, including perineal discomfort. It found that significantly fewer women in the intensive PFME group (9%) reported experiencing perineal pain in the previous week than in the control group (13%), although there were no differences in dyspareunia or how early intercourse had been resumed. PFME are generally taught to prevent or treat stress incontinence, as described in the guideline on Urinary Problems, but the findings of the above study suggest it also may help relieve perineal pain.

## Removal of suture material

No studies have assessed the impact on perineal pain of removing suture material, either because the suture is 'tight' or because of friction from a knot in the material. Anecdotal experience does, however, suggest that selective removal of material may reduce perineal discomfort. In the trial by Kettle and colleagues (2002) referred to earlier, use of polyglactin 910 suture material resulted in less need to remove suture material in the first 3 months.

## Haematoma

A haematoma may occur following trauma to the perineum, inadequate suturing of perineal trauma or traumatic vaginal delivery including shoulder dystocia. Haematomas are rare among the postnatal population, one clinical review reporting an incidence of between 1 in 500 to 1 in 900 (Ridgway 1995). The site of the haematoma can be vulvar, vaginal or subperitoneal (Gross et al 1987). Onset can occur immediately following delivery, but delayed onset can occur days or even weeks after the birth, possibly as a consequence of failure to recognise a haematoma prior to hospital discharge.

Haematomas are extremely painful and prompt identification and management are essential. Incision and drainage may be required to alleviate symptoms but this will depend on the severity and extent of the haematoma (Propst & Thorp 1998). As this is an acute symptom, immediate referral should be made to the GP or obstetric unit.

## Management: dyspareunia

There is much less research evidence on the management of postpartum dyspareunia. In the trial by Sleep & Grant (1987) described above, of routine versus intensive pelvic floor exercises, there was no difference in the reported prevalence of dyspareunia at 3 months. Nor was there any difference in subsequent dyspareunia or in the earlier resumption of intercourse between the groups in the trial of bath additives (Sleep & Grant 1988b).

Women who have had perineal trauma could be informed that they may find resumption of intercourse painful, as knowledge of this may provide reassurance that they are not 'abnormal'. If women do find intercourse painful, lubricating gel may ease soreness on penetration, particularly when intercourse is first attempted. In the NCT survey by Greenshields & Hulme (1993), it was reported that some women found that vaginal lubrication, oils or gels rubbed into the perineum, or relaxation techniques, eased pain during intercourse. Women who are breastfeeding could be advised of this, as they may be more likely to experience vaginal dryness (Barrett et al 2000). Expert advice suggests that a specialist clinic can be of benefit in treatment of women who experience painful intercourse, although further research on the management of this problem after childbirth is required.

## SUMMARY OF THE EVIDENCE USED IN THIS GUIDELINE

- Observational studies and data from trials have shown that short-term and longer term perineal pain and dyspareunia are common symptoms after childbirth.

- Evidence from various types of studies indicates that women who have instrumental deliveries have more perineal pain and dyspareunia than with other forms of delivery, but the independent effects of mode of delivery and type of perineal trauma are difficult to separate.

- Evidence from a systematic review has shown that restricted compared with liberal episiotomy policies do not differ in relation to perineal pain or dyspareunia but there are other adverse outcomes indicating that a routine episiotomy policy could not be supported.

- Evidence from a systematic review has shown that the use of synthetic materials to repair perineal trauma results in less pain than the use of catgut.

- Evidence from one randomised controlled trial showed that the use of rapidly absorbed polyglactin 910 material resulted in less need to remove suture material within the first 3 months of the birth.

- Evidence from a systematic review has shown that the use of a continuous subcuticular suturing technique is associated with less short-term pain than interrupted sutures, but further evidence is required on longer term pain and dyspareunia.

- One large randomised controlled trial found a two-stage procedure of perineal repair, with the skin not sutured, to be associated with a small reduction in dyspareunia at 3 months although there was no difference in perineal pain.

- Further research is required to assess the effects of not suturing second-degree perineal tears.

- One large randomised controlled trial showed that vaginal delivery with 'hands on' compared with 'hands poised' was associated with less short-term perineal pain but there were no longer term differences.

- Randomised controlled trials and observational studies of various treatments for postpartum perineal pain and dyspareunia show that evidence of long term benefit is sparse.

- Evidence to support the use of topically applied anaesthetics is not robust, and further trials are required.

## WHAT TO DO

### Perineal pain – General advice

- Most women who have delivered vaginally will have some degree of perineal discomfort initially, so general advice is appropriate for most.
  Acknowledgement that perineal pain is common, and that the trauma will heal in time, may help relieve any anxiety.
- Note delivery details. Observe perineum if possible, to obtain a 'baseline' recording. Bruising, oedema, inflammation or gaping in the wound edges should be noted.
- NICE (2006) recommends that women should be asked at each subsequent contact if they have any concerns about the healing of their perineum.
- Regular analgesia (paracetamol) can be taken to relieve discomfort.
  If paracetamol is ineffective, referral for oral or rectal NSAID (unless contraindicated) should be made, particularly for women with a large tear or extended episiotomy. Medication that can cause constipation (i.e. co-codamol) should be avoided.

- Dietary advice to avoid constipation should be given (refer to guideline on Bowel Problems), particularly if there is a large tear or extended episiotomy, as straining may increase perineal pain.
- Perineal hygiene should be discussed as appropriate. Sanitary pads should be changed frequently, washing hands before and after, and daily bathing and showering will help to keep the perineal area clean.

## Management

- Examine the perineum to detect signs of possible infection, oedema or inadequate repair. Ask for a description of type of pain (e.g. sharp or burning), whether it follows a particular activity (e.g. when micturating or defaecating) and if there is offensive vaginal loss. This information may aid 'diagnosis' of the problem and enable more effective care/advice.
- Application of ice packs or cooling gel pads may provide short-term pain relief
- Some women find bathing soothing, but advise that bath additives will not aid healing.
- There is no trial evidence that alternative therapies have any effect, but anecdotal evidence suggests some women find benefit. Alternative remedies should only be used if the midwife or woman is experienced in their application.
- If a perineal wound infection is suspected, a swab should be taken and the woman referred (urgent action). Ensure adequate analgesia and stress the importance of hygiene to prevent spread of infection. A woman may also have complained of an offensive loss, which may be a result of an infected perineal wound. If offensive loss is reported but not associated with a wound infection, refer to guideline on Endometritis and Abnormal Blood Loss for management of offensive lochia.
- If a suture has become too tight and requires removal, this should be done with sterile scissors, not stitch cutters. The knot should be cut, not pulled through the skin. This may ease discomfort immediately and reduce associated swelling/oedema.
- If there is discomfort related to passing urine or frequency of micturition, exclude UTI (refer to guideline on Urinary Problems). Check the woman's temperature. If she is pyrexial and pain is experienced during micturition, take an MSU and refer (urgent action). If there are symptoms of stress incontinence, refer to guideline on Urinary Problems, as it is possible that involuntary loss of urine may irritate perineal trauma.
- If the perineum is bruised, assess extent of bruising compared with baseline observation. If bruising has not increased, advise woman to continue to take analgesia. Bathing may provide temporary relief. If bruising site is extended and perineal skin is tense, shiny and hard, there may be a haematoma and the woman should be referred (urgent action).
- Following diagnosis of the problem, visits should be planned to assess progress once appropriate advice and/or treatment have been given.

## Dyspareunia – General advice

All women should be given advice about contraception and resumption of intercourse preferably within 2–3 weeks of delivery when some women will resume intercourse. Women who have had perineal trauma should be informed that intercourse may be painful at first, as this may reassure them that they are not 'abnormal'.

### Management

- If the woman reports painful intercourse, although there is a lack of research evidence on effective management, anecdotal evidence suggests that use of a water-based lubricant gel may ease discomfort. This information is particularly important for breastfeeding women, who may be more likely to experience vaginal dryness.
- If the woman had any perineal trauma, observe (if possible) for signs of inadequate repair (sometimes trauma is not correctly anatomically approximated) or scarring of suture line, which could result in dyspareunia. If this is indicated, the woman should be advised and referred (non-urgent action).
- Anecdotal evidence is available on the benefit of oils and gels rubbed into the perineum to ease discomfort during intercourse, but these should only be recommended if the woman or the midwife has experience of using alternative therapies.
- Women who express anxieties about resuming sexual intercourse may be concerned about the possibility of another pregnancy. If so, contraception should be discussed and referral to the GP or to a family planning clinic made to decide on the most suitable method.
- If appropriate, discuss with the woman and/or her partner that enthusiasm for a sexual relationship may be reduced for a period of time after childbirth.
- If dyspareunia persists and the woman feels it is a problem, she should be referred (non-urgent action).

## SUMMARY GUIDELINE

# Perineal pain and dyspareunia

## Initial assessment

- Most women who have had a vaginal delivery will have some perineal discomfort
- Obtain baseline observation of perineum to assess bruising, extent of trauma and healing
- If third-degree tear, refer to guideline on Bowel Problems for advice on preventing constipation
- Give general advice as appropriate

## Urgent action is required if:

- Suspected perineal wound infection
- Suspected vulval haematoma

## General advice

- Reassure that perineal pain is common
- Advise on analgesia (paracetamol) if needed. Consider referral for oral or rectal NSAID medication (non-urgent action)
- Advise on perineal hygiene
- Discuss benefits of temporary pain relief from using gel pads, ice packs and bathing
- Ask at each contact about concerns about perineal healing
- Reassure that it is not abnormal for intercourse after childbirth to be uncomfortable and that lubricant gel may ease soreness

# What to do

## Persistent perineal pain

- Assess condition of perineum and the progress of healing
- Explore nature of pain and exclude other possible causes, e.g. UTI
- Ensure that analgesia is effective
- If bruising is severe, exclude haematoma – if present, refer (urgent action)
- If infection suspected, take swab and refer (urgent action)
- Remove any tight sutures with sterile scissors as this may ease pain
- Advise that bathing may ease symptoms temporarily, but will not aid healing
- Review progress at each subsequent contact

## Dyspareunia

- Check for inadequate perineal repair, persistent perineal trauma or scarring. If present, referral should be made (non-urgent action)
- Stress that use of lubricant gel may ease soreness on penetration
- Ensure contraception is not a concern
- Reassure that many couples find that enthusiasm for intercourse is reduced for a time after childbirth
- Referral should be made if perineal pain or dyspareunia continues to be a problem

# References

Barrett G, Pendry E, Peacock J et al 1998 Sexual function after childbirth: women's experiences, persistent morbidity and lack of professional recognition (letter). Br J Obstet Gynaecol 105: 242-244

Barrett G, Pendry E, Peacock J et al 2000 Women's sexual health after childbirth. Br J Obstet Gynaecol 107(2): 186-195

Binder A, Hodge G, Greenwood A et al 1985 Is therapeutic ultrasound effective in the treatment of soft tissue lesions? BMJ 290: 512-514

Brown S, Lumley J 1998 Changing childbirth: lessons from an Australian survey of 1336 women. Br J Obstet Gynaecol 105(2): 143-155

Buhling KJ, Schmidt S, Robinson JN et al 2006 Rate of dyspareunia after delivery in primiparae according to mode of delivery. Eur J Obstet Reprod Biol 124(1): 42-46

Carroli G, Belizan J, Stamp G 2000 Episiotomy for vaginal birth. Cochrane Database of Systematic Reviews, Issue 1

Dale A, Cornwell S 1994 The role of lavender oil in relieving perineal discomfort following childbirth: a blind randomized clinical trial. J Adv Nurs 19(1): 89-96

Fleming VEM, Hagen S, Niven C 2003 Does perineal suturing make a difference? The SUNS trial. Br J Obstet Gynaecol 110: 684-689

Glazener CMA 1997 Sexual function after childbirth: women's experiences, persistent morbidity and lack of professional recognition. Br J Obstet Gynaecol 104: 330-335

Glazener CMA 1998 Sexual function after childbirth (letter). Br J Obstet Gynaecol 105: 241-248

Glazener C, Abdalla M, Stroud P et al 1995 Postnatal maternal morbidity: extent, causes, prevention and treatment. Br J Obstet Gynaecol 102: 282-287

Gordon B, Mackrodt C, Fern E et al 1998 The Ipswich Childbirth Study:1. A randomised evaluation of two stage postpartum perineal repair leaving the skin unsutured. Br J Obstet Gynaecol 105(4): 435-440

Greenshields W, Hulme H 1993 The perineum in childbirth. A survey of women's experiences and midwives practices. National Childbirth Trust, London

Griffiths A, Watermeyer S, Sidhu K et al 2006 Female genital tract morbidity and sexual function following vaginal delivery or lower segment caesarean section. J Obstet Gynecol 26(7): 645-649

Gross ST, Shime J, Farine D 1987 Shoulder dystocia: predictors and outcome. A five year review. Am J Obstet Gynecol 156: 334-336

Hay-Smith EJC 2000 Therapeutic ultrasound for postpartum perineal pain and dyspareunia. Cochrane Database of Systematic Reviews, Issue 3

Hedayati H, Parsons J, Crowther CA 2003 Rectal analgesia for pain from perineal trauma following childbirth. Cochrane Database of Systematic Reviews, Issue 3

Hedayati H, Parsons J, Crowther CA 2005 Topically applied anaesthetics for treating perineal pain after childbirth. Cochrane Database of Systematic Reviews, Issue 2

Johanson RB, Rice C, Doyle M et al 1993 A randomised prospective study comparing the new vacuum extractor policy with forceps delivery. Br J Obstet Gynaecol 100: 524-530

Kettle C, Johanson RB 1999 Absorbable synthetic versus catgut suture material for perineal repair. Cochrane Database of Systematic Reviews, Issue 3

Kettle C, Hills RK, Jones P et al 2002 Continuous versus interrupted perineal repair with standard or rapidly absorbed sutures after spontaneous vaginal birth: a randomised controlled trial. Lancet 359(9325): 2217

Kettle C, Hills RK, Ismail KMK Continuous versus interrupted sutures for repair of episiotomy or second degree tears. Cochrane Database of Systematic Reviews 2007, Issue 4

Klein MC, Gauthier RJ, Robbins JM et al 1994 Relationship of episiotomy to perineal trauma and morbidity, sexual dysfunction and pelvic floor relaxation. Am J Obstet Gynecol 171(3): 591-598

Lundquist M, Olsson A, Nissen E et al 2000 Is it necessary to suture all lacerations after a vaginal delivery? Birth 27: 79-85

Macarthur AJ, Macarthur C 2004 Incidence, severity and determinants of perineal pain after vaginal delivery: a prospective cohort study. Am J Obstet Gynecol 191(4): 1199-1204

McCandlish R 2001 Perineal trauma: prevention and treatment. J Midwifery Women's Health 46(6): 396-401

McCandlish R, Bowler U, van Asten H et al 1998 A randomised controlled trial of care of the perineum during second stage of normal labour. Br J Obstet Gynaecol 105(12): 1262-1272

Metcalfe A, Bick D, Tohill S et al 2006 A prospective cohort study of repair and non-repair of second-degree perineal trauma: results and issues for future research. Evidence-Based Midwifery 4(2): 60-64

National Institute for Health and Clinical Excellence 2006 Postnatal Care: Routine postnatal care of women and their babies. NICE Clinical Guidelines 37

Propst AM, Thorp JM Jr 1998 Traumatic vulvar hematomas: conservative versus surgical management. South Med J 91(2): 144-146

Ramler D, Roberts J 1986 A comparison of cold and warm sitz baths for relief of postpartum perineal pain. JOGNN 15: 471-474

Ridgway L 1995 Puerperal emergency. Vaginal and vulvar haematomas. Obstet Gynecol Clin North Am 275-282

Signorello LB, Harlow BL, Chekos AK et al 2001 Postpartum sexual functioning and its relationship to perineal trauma: a retrospective cohort study of primiparous women. Am J Obstet Gynecol 184(5): 881-888

Sleep J 1990 Postnatal perineal care. In: Alexander J, Levy V, Roch S (eds) Postnatal care: a research based approach. Macmillan, London

Sleep J 1995 Postnatal perineal care revisited. In: Alexander J, Levy V, Roch S (eds) Aspects of midwifery practice. A research based approach. Macmillan, London

Sleep J, Grant A 1987 Pelvic floor exercises in postnatal care – the report of a randomised controlled trial to compare an intensive exercise regimen with the programme in current use. Midwifery 3: 158 164

Sleep J, Grant A 1988a The relief of perineal pain following childbirth: a survey of midwifery practice. Midwifery 4: 118-122

Sleep J, Grant A 1988b Effects of salt and savlon bath concentrate postpartum. Nursing Times 84(21): 55-57

Sleep J, Grant A, Garcia J et al 1984 West Berkshire perineal management trial. BMJ 289: 587-590

Steen M, Cooper K 1997 A tool for assessing perineal trauma. J Wound Care 6(9): 432-436

Steen M, Cooper K, Marchant P et al 2000 A randomised controlled trial to compare the effectiveness of icepacks and Epifoam with cooling maternity gel pads at alleviating postnatal perineal trauma. Midwifery 16: 48-55

# Chapter 3

# Caesarean section wound care and pain relief

## INTRODUCTION

In addition to the other changes of the postpartum period, women who have had their baby delivered by caesarean section have an abdominal wound which requires monitoring and care. Common infections following caesarean section include urinary tract infection (UTI), endometritis and wound infection (Leigh et al 1990). Urinary tract infection and endometritis are discussed in the guideline on Urinary Problems and the guideline on Endometritis and Abnormal Blood Loss respectively, and the main issues in this guideline are wound infection and pain management.

The literature relating to wound care presented in this guideline refers specifically to caesarean section, but the principles of care can be applied to a postpartum sterilisation wound.

### Caesarean section rates

The number of caesarean sections performed in the UK and other developed countries has increased steadily over the past 20 years. The most recent Department of Health maternity statistics bulletin reported that 22.7% of all deliveries in England and Wales were by caesarean section during the period 2003–04 (Department of Health 2005). This rate had increased from 18.2% in 1994–95, having been 10.4% in 1985. The National Sentinel Caesarean Section Audit found that the caesarean section rate (CSR) in the UK increased with maternal age and was higher in black African or black

Caribbean women compared to white women (Thomas & Paranjothy 2001). Previous surveys of caesarean section rates found considerable variation between hospitals in England and Wales, with a range from 6.2% to 21.5% (Francome et al 1993), and that women who attended teaching hospitals were more likely to have a caesarean section than women in other hospitals, but there was also variation in rates between teaching hospitals (Savage & Francome 1993).

The trend towards earlier postnatal discharge from hospital for women delivered vaginally has also been seen following caesarean section. The average hospital stay following caesarean section in 2003–04 was between 3 and 4 days, having been between 4 and 5 days during the 6-year period up to 1994–95 (Department of Health 1997), and 8 days in a large national study conducted in 1983 (Moir-Bussy et al 1984). Only one randomised controlled trial (RCT) included in the Cochrane review of early postnatal discharge (Brown et al 2002) had a study population of 162 US women who had (unplanned) caesarean section (Brooten et al 1994). Outcomes were compared between those who were discharged early and those randomised to usual hospital discharge. The 61 women in the early discharge group were sent home a mean of 30.3 hours earlier and were significantly more satisfied with care than the usual care group.

It is likely that all but the most immediate requirements for postoperative care of the woman and her wound will be in the community and more complications and infections will be diagnosed there (Beattie et al 1994). Midwives in the community will therefore continue to see an increasing number of women who have had a caesarean section, and at an earlier stage of their postoperative course.

## IMMEDIATE CARE AFTER CAESAREAN SECTION

A clinical guideline for caesarean section commissioned by National Institute for Health and Clinical Excellence published in 2004 covers aspects of care of the woman and of the baby up to hospital discharge (National Co-ordinating Centre for Women's and Children's Health 2004). This guideline is complementary to the NICE postnatal guideline (NICE 2006) which provides guidance on routine community care of healthy women and their babies, including after caesarean section.

## WOUND INFECTION FOLLOWING CAESAREAN SECTION

### Definition

There is no universally agreed definition of wound infection following caesarean section. Signs of inflammation such as erythema and induration are not specific to infection and irritation from the suture material can cause similar appearances. It is possible that serous discharge from the wound may occur without infection but infection is likely when such discharge is purulent. Additional evidence of infection, in the form of positive bacteriological culture in material from the wound, is not always obtained. Studies vary in the criteria used to classify the wound as infected. The definition used in the *National Survey of Infection in Hospitals* published in 1981 was that of inflammation or discharge of pus and positive bacteriological culture (Meers 1981). This was the definition used in a national survey of wound infection following caesarean section in 1984 (Moir-Bussy et al 1984). It was also the basis for the definition used in a prospective study following caesarean section by Parrott et al (1989), but in this study a wound swab or pus sample was taken for bacteriological culture from all patients with signs of wound infection or with postoperative pyrexia. A positive culture was accepted as evidence of wound infection with or without signs of inflammation or sepsis. In another study of postcaesarean women, the diagnosis was made on clinical features alone (Pirwany & Mahmood 1997). Leigh et al (1990) included cases with either clinical or bacteriological findings of infection. In one survey of general surgical patients, follow-up extended into the community, and the definition of wound infection included cases where antibiotics were used to treat a previously uninfected but inflamed wound (Weigelt et al 1992).

## Frequency of occurrence

Moir-Bussy et al (1984) undertook the first major prospective study of the incidence of wound infection after caesarean section in the UK. The method of selection of the 31 participating hospitals is not entirely clear so some reservations about generalisability of the findings remain. Survey questionnaires were completed for 2370 women having a section over a 12-week period in 1983. An overall infection rate of 6% (n = 141) was reported, with a range of zero to 20.5% between hospitals. In the study, definitions of classification terms used were clear but there is no evidence that objectivity, consistency and completeness between and within centres were achieved. Indeed, although the definition of wound infection used was inflammation or sepsis and a positive bacteriological culture in material taken from the wound, not all centres involved in the study collected swabs for culture on all women with clinical presentation. Culture from inflamed wounds was positive in 80% of cases and, in a later paper, the team suggest that if this rate were applied to the wounds recorded as inflamed but not cultured, the infection rate would have been 14% (Thompson et al 1987).

This study demonstrates the difficulty arising from the lack of a universal method of classifying wounds as infected when determining its incidence. Estimates of wound infection rates from studies which required positive bacteriological culture in the classification are: 4.1% (Hawrylyshyn et al 1981) and 7% (Hillan 1995). The rate was 11.3% from the study where wound infection was classified on positive culture with or without clinical evidence of inflammation or sepsis (Parrot et al 1989).

Higher rates were reported when clinical findings alone were taken as evidence of infection in the absence of a positive bacterial culture, with rates of between 15.8% and 29.2% (Henderson & Love 1995, Leigh et al 1990). The wound infection rate was 25.3% in Beattie et al's (1994) study which, in addition to clinical or bacteriological evidence, included cases where antibiotics were prescribed for wound infection without the study team having any further information of the clinical features. Follow-up in this study was also extended beyond discharge from hospital which will further inflate the rate. In the report of a self-completion questionnaire survey at 3 months postpartum, of 444 women who had had a caesarean section, 121 (27%) reported having had a wound infection at some point (Hillan 1992). It seems that only for 43 of these were antibiotics prescribed.

The trend is for rates to be higher when the diagnosis is made without requiring positive culture. Estimates based on positive culture alone are also subject to error. In the Moir-Bussy survey, *Staphylococcus albus* was the commonest organism cultured (Moir-Bussy et al 1984). The authors themselves acknowledge that this organism is an unlikely pathogen. If the cases where this was the sole organism cultured were removed from the numerator, the wound infection rate would have been 4.5% rather than 6%, but many of the cases where this was the sole organism cultured had clinical evidence of a wound infection. Classification for study purposes may differ from routine management, however, and in practice antibiotic therapy may well be instituted without culturing the pus or taking a swab of an inflamed wound.

As noted earlier, wound infection rates differed with time in Leigh et al's study of 202 women having caesarean sections in 1985 and 196 women in 1987 (Leigh et al 1990). All women in this observational study had their wounds assessed daily (excluding weekends) by the study laboratory nurse until discharge from hospital. Swabs were taken from all inflamed wounds, whether or not there was discharge from the wound. Wound infections were classified into two groups: clinical, where there was inflammation and discharge but culture did not show any pathogenic bacteria; and bacteriological, where recognised pathogens were present. The incidence of clinical wound infection was 20% in 1985 and 15.8% in 1987, but bacteriologically proven infections were 12.5% and 5.1% respectively. Since the same methodology was used for each series, with no significant difference in the caesarean section rate, it is surprising that the reported incidence of wound infection is so different. No explanations are offered by the authors. Other audits of different time periods have largely endeavoured to show an effect of antibiotic prophylaxis on infection rate (Nice et al 1996, Pirwany & Mahmood 1997).

## Presentation

The onset of wound infection following caesarean section has been described between the first and 15th postoperative day, most commonly manifested on day 4 or 5 (Leigh et al 1990, Moir-Bussy et al 1984). Since some women will not develop the infection until after discharge from hospital, the true incidence of wound infection is probably even higher than that reported in these studies. The majority of studies of wound infections were hospital-based retrospective chart reviews, leaving little scope for follow-up to identify infections after discharge. In almost all cases surveillance was limited to the hospital inpatient stay and although in one study observation was stated to be for 6 weeks, no indication was given of the completeness of hospital case-notes regarding the period following discharge (Pirwany & Mahmood 1997). Hulton et al (1992) showed that the overall rates of infection following caesarean section were underestimates if based on inpatient data alone. They ascertained the number of infections which occurred following discharge by writing to the woman's surgeon at 6 weeks postpartum. The wound infection rate rose from 0.3% in 318 women who had caesarean sections in the 5-month period before this postdischarge method of ascertainment to 3.9% in the 5-month period after it was initiated (n = 500).

Three studies identified women prospectively (Beattie et al 1994, Nice et al 1996, Parrot et al 1989) but in one, surveillance was completed on day 6 post section (Parrot et al 1989). Nice et al's study (1996) of 628 postsection women was prospective and follow-up was continued after discharge by the community midwife but surveillance stopped at the 10th postoperative day. Beattie et al (1994) also identified 428 women prospectively and followed them up beyond hospital discharge but it is not stated for how long. Of the 83 wound infections diagnosed in the 328 women on whom the results are based, 30 (36.2%) were diagnosed after discharge from hospital.

It is likely, however, that findings from the Weigelt et al (1992) general surgical wound surveillance programme are paralleled for caesarean section patients. For 30 days after surgery the programme followed 16,453 consecutive patients operated on in various surgical specialties in Dallas, Texas, during a 6-year period between 1983 and 1989. Surveillance was by infection control practitioners (ICPs) and clinic nurses instructed in wound evaluation by the ICPs. Surgeons were not involved with the classification of wounds to reduce any observer bias. Of all surgical wound infections that were diagnosed, 35% (516) first became apparent after discharge from hospital. Less than half (47%) of wound infections were manifest by the seventh postoperative day, 78% were diagnosed by day 14 and 90% by day 21. A small number of infections continued to be first diagnosed between days 21 and 30.

Of the wounds that did become infected, those which occurred in obese patients were more likely to be first diagnosed after discharge rather than in hospital.

As discussed previously, there is no standard definition of what constitutes a wound infection, but the signs and symptoms suggestive of wound infection have been described above: pyrexia, localised pain and erythema, local oedema (induration), excess exudate, pus and offensive odour (Meers 1981, Morrison 1992). The diagnosis will therefore be made on the basis of patient reporting of pain, discharge, separation or fever and by visual inspection of the wound.

If a wound infection is suspected, a swab should be taken for identification of the organism and antibiotic sensitivity testing. The sample should be collected before the wound is cleaned, avoiding the surrounding skin, which may be colonised by different organisms from the one(s) causing the wound infection (Dealey 1994).

Apart from the need to relieve pain and deal with discharge, the concern with any wound infection is the possibility of breakdown. Dehiscence (separation of the wound edges) may be superficial, involving only the skin layer, or may extend to the deep layers. In severe cases there may be protrusion of the abdominal cavity contents (burst abdomen).

Most caesarean sections are performed using a Pfannenstiel skin and lower uterine segment incisions. In a series of 1300 caesarean sections, the majority of which were performed through Pfannenstiel incisions, none dehisced, although six cases of dehiscence occurred in the series following midline incisions (Donald 1979). Denominators for these figures were not quoted. Where the incision is midline, there is a greater risk of both dehiscence and herniation, but no published evidence of actual rates of occurrence following caesarean section were found. In abdominal laparotomy incisions in general surgical patients, the rate of burst abdomen (complete dehiscence) is of the order of 1–2% (Ausobsky et al 1985, Bucknall 1983).

Due to these concerns, women in whom wound infection is detected while inpatients are often kept under observation for longer. In the Moir-Bussy study (1984) average inpatient stay increased by 2 days for those who developed postcaesarean wound infection in hospital. The average stay for a woman who did not develop a wound infection in their study was 8 days. In the Canadian study by Henderson & Love (1995), the mean duration of hospital stay was increased in women with wound infection by 0.8 days in first section cases (from a mean of 5.9) and by 0.4 days in second or more sections (from a mean of 5.5 days). Mean stay was inflated more by certain other types of postcaesarean infection, but because of its relative frequency, wound infection had the greatest overall impact on extra bed days required.

As stated earlier, follow-up data on caesarean section patients after discharge from hospital are scarce. Of 30 women in Beattie's survey who had a wound infection diagnosed after discharge from hospital, two required readmission (Beattie et al 1994). No details are given of the indication or of subsequent treatment requirements.

## Risk factors

In relation to *all* infectious morbidity following caesarean section (endometritis, urinary tract infection, wound infection, etc.), associations with many factors have been suggested (Hawrylyshyn et al 1981, Smail & Hofmeyr 2002). There is less evidence relating to the risk factors specific to wound infection. There are no systematic reviews of the evidence and, as has been discussed, most of the studies are retrospective case-note reviews relating only to complications identified during the inpatient period.

Using simple univariate comparisons between groups of patients in their survey, Moir-Bussy et al (1984) suggested that the following were statistically significant risk factors for wound infection following caesarean section: higher weight/height ratio (as recorded in early pregnancy); higher numbers of vaginal examinations during labour; longer duration of labour; not being nursed in a ward where only caesarean section patients were nursed; alcoholic chlorhexidine not being used for skin preparation preoperatively; the skin incision being paramedian or midline rather than Pfannenstiel; having a drain of any sort; skin closure issues; having a plastic dressing rather than a material one; and being delivered by section in a unit where less than 50 caesarean sections were performed over the 12-week period of the survey (Moir-Bussy et al 1984).

Factors also considered in the Moir-Bussy survey, but found *not* to be statistically significant included: social class (proportionately more women from social classes IV and V were affected, but this difference was not statistically significant); emergency versus elective caesarean; duration of ruptured membranes; epidural or general anaesthesia; anaemia; and being delivered in a teaching or non-teaching hospital.

In their prospective study of 428 women who had a caesarean section, Beattie et al (1994) also described a link between obesity and wound infection, although they used last recorded weight as the index of obesity. Complete data were only available for 76.6% (n = 328) of the population in this study, and 44.2% of these women had some form of antibiotic prophylaxis. The study also showed a statistically significant, negative association between maternal age and wound infection but failed to show a statistically significant association between number of vaginal examinations and wound infection. Although there was a proportionately higher rate of infection for patients who had a drain inserted at the operation, this was not statistically significant. The authors state that a multivariate analysis method was used and the protective effect of prophylactic antibiotics was very strong so that demonstration of independent effects of other factors may be prohibited.

In general, studies have not attempted to clarify whether postoperative factors beyond the first day influence development of infection in the wound.

In a retrospective chart review of 1335 caesarean section cases between 1985 and 1988, Henderson & Love (1995) found that incisional wound infection was higher in first caesarean sections than in repeat sections, and was higher in elective section compared to emergency. Possible explanations suggested for this were decreased use of prophylactic antibiotics in elective sections or that the interval between preoperative shaving and surgery in elective section may predispose to wound infection. Leigh et al (1990) found a higher rate of bacteriologically confirmed infections after elective caesarean section, but no difference for clinical infection.

## Antibiotic prophylaxis

The evidence from 66 randomised controlled trials was examined in a systematic review undertaken to determine whether prophylactic antibiotic treatment given to women undergoing caesarean section decreased the incidence of febrile morbidity, wound and other infections, or serious infectious complications (Smaill & Hofmeyr 2002). The review included trials that compared *any* prophylactic antibiotic regimen with placebo or no treatment. The lack of consistent application of a standard definition for wound infection (and endometritis) was noted in the background to the review and, in the trials, endometritis and wound infection were usually defined clinically, without bacteriological confirmation.

The main outcome measure reported was all infectious morbidity and the findings of the review were that 'the use of prophylactic antibiotics at caesarean section resulted in a major, clinically important and statistically significant decrease in the incidence of fever, endometritis, wound infection, urinary tract infection and serious infection after caesarean section'. Only for endometritis was a measure of effect given, with its rate of occurrence reduced by 73% (95% confidence interval (CI) 0.68–0.77) for all women undergoing the procedure. Prior to the review it was controversial whether prophylaxis should be reserved for cases in which the risk of infection was higher, but the size of the reduction in endometritis was consistent even when elective and non-elective sections were considered separately.

Hospital stay was reduced by 0.34 days (95% CI 0.10–0.51) in those who received prophylaxis, but there was too little information in general to allow costs of the two strategies to be compared.

In the data from trials where elective caesarean sections were identified, no statistically significant reduction in wound or urinary tract infection was seen with prophylaxis in this group. Although this could be because the trials were too small, even collectively, to show a positive effect, the reviewers had to conclude that while prophylaxis is recommended based on the reduction in endometritis, the rate of wound infections following elective caesarean section may not be seen to fall.

The review recommended that all units should have a policy of administering prophylactic antibiotics at caesarean section. A policy of not treating all women undergoing caesarean should only be considered in units that have prospectively confirmed a low rate of infection in women using methods where follow-up was long enough to include late complications.

## Management

There are no trials examining wound management in an obstetric population. However, a randomised trial of 1202 general surgery postoperative patients found that removing the dressing after the first 24 postoperative hours had several advantages (Chrintz et al 1989). Wounds can be easily examined for early signs of complications; time and materials necessary for the renewal of wound dressings are reduced; personal hygiene is easier to carry out without a wound dressing. A sutured wound is not a contraindication to washing or showering after 24 hours. In this study there was no increase in the incidence of infection in wounds, which were left uncovered after 24 hours. There will be circumstances when a dressing is required beyond this time, e.g. if there is exudate from a wound infection.

The aims of applying dressings to an infected wound are to absorb secretions and to protect the wound from injury and bacterial contamination. There is a wide variety of dressings available, making choice difficult. No single dressing is suitable for all wounds (Morrison 1992), and each wound should be assessed individually and comprehensively (Tallon 1996). Assessment should include the condition of the wound; the presence or absence of exudate; the depth of the wound; and the time available to visit the patient at home to dress the wound. The 'ideal' wound dressing is described as having the following properties: control of moisture content, gaseous permeability, no/low adherence, being impermeable to bacteria, thermal properties, protection of the wound from further trauma, being non-toxic and non-allergenic (Dealey 1994, Morrison 1992, Thomas 1990).

There is a lack of trial evidence to support any particular type of dressing specific to infected abdominal surgical wounds. Some health trusts have developed their own wound management policies.

No studies describing the indications for systemic antibiotics were found. In Hillan's self-completion survey of women post caesarean section, approximately 7% of those who reported having had a wound infection had antibiotics prescribed for this infection (Hillan 1992). In women who develop a wound infection, it is probably advisable to find out which specific antibiotic was given prophylactically, especially if treating them without bacteriological confirmation, as it may influence the choice of any antibiotic given.

Obesity is a risk factor for wound infection and, although there is no evidence of effective ways of improving risk, a higher index of suspicion should be retained in obese women post caesarean section. It is likely that women will be tentative in exposure of the wound when washing. Although there is no trial evidence to support the recommendation, it seems sensible to discuss the necessity, when washing, of raising any skinfolds which occlude the wound when sitting or standing.

Adherence to correct handwashing techniques and general hygiene measures by health professionals and by the woman herself (Bell & Fenton 1993) is vital.

If surveillance is not continued until 21 days after surgery, the woman should be advised of the ongoing possibility of infection and whom she should contact with any problem.

## PAIN RELIEF IN THE IMMEDIATE POSTOPERATIVE PERIOD

### Wound pain

Few studies have described the occurrence of pain in the postpartum period. An Aberdeen survey of postnatal pain experienced by 198 postpartum women included 26 women delivered by caesarean section (Dewan et al 1993). The women were questioned about any pain – uterine cramps, perineal or abdominal wound, breast, etc. – experienced in the previous 12 hours. They were surveyed on days 1, 2 and 4 (if still in hospital). Overall, 95% of the women reported at least one type of pain on the first day after delivery, but by the fourth day most had settled. For the women who had had a caesarean, the most important source of pain was their wound and on day 4, 73% still had wound pain.

The mainstay of analgesia in the immediate postoperative period has been opioid-based drugs administered by injection. These may cause drowsiness, nausea and respiratory depression, thus reducing the woman's ability to care for her baby. Some trials comparing the efficacy of perioperative interventions in reducing pain after caesarean section have been reported.

Non-steroidal anti-inflammatory drugs (NSAIDs) have been used in the treatment of rheumatic disease for over 25 years, and during the past 10 years have become more commonly used to treat postoperative pain. Side-effects are rare but the usual contraindications apply: bleeding disturbances, allergy or previous marked side-effects to NSAIDs, asthma, previous gastrointestinal ulceration, atopia or diabetes, etc. Most NSAIDs do increase bleeding time slightly, and they may inhibit contractions of the pregnant uterus. Given in large doses, NSAIDs can cause premature closure of the ductus arteriosus.

Publications on the use of NSAIDs in the relief of postcaesarean section pain have concentrated largely on the the first 48 hours following surgery (Bush et al 1992, Dennis et al 1995, Rorarius et al 1993). Available papers therefore relate to relief of intense pain and the use of stronger NSAIDs, such as diclofenac. The measures of outcome often include whether the amount of opioid (administered intramuscularly or via a patient-controlled analgesia system (PCA)) required is reduced or delayed.

In a double-blind randomised controlled trial, Bush et al (1992) evaluated the use of a single dose of intramuscular diclofenac (an NSAID) after elective caesarean section under general anaesthesia. The outcome measure used was the patient's postoperative requirement for opioid analgesia (papaveretum) by a PCA system. Mean opioid consumption in the diclofenac group was significantly lower than for the control group during the first 18 hours (61.4 mg vs 91.4 mg, $p < 0.05$). The authors also found that equal or superior analgesia was achieved within the first 6 hours with less sedation in the diclofenac group. This was a small study; 23 women were allocated to receive diclofenac 75 mg, and 25 had an equal volume of normal saline but the findings were consistent with previous work showing a similar effect following some forms of abdominal surgery (hysterectomy) though not others (cholecystectomy).

In a Finnish study, Rorarius et al (1993) compared the effects of intravenous infusions of diclofenac 150 mg (n = 29) and ketoprofen 200 mg (n = 30) in a randomised controlled trial of 90 women who had elective caesarean section under spinal or epidural block. A control group (n = 30) received an infusion of normal saline. Requirement for postoperative opioids was decreased by 40% in women receiving NSAIDs. One of the women who received diclofenac developed uterine atony requiring intravenous uterine stimulatants to be administered. It was the author's view that the dosage of diclofenac received was insufficient to have caused this problem but the infusion was stopped as initial treatment failed to reverse the atonic uterus.

Rectal diclofenac 100 mg was assessed after elective caesarean section using spinal hyperbaric bupivacaine and spinal morphine in a double-blind randomised placebo-controlled trial (Dennis et al 1995). Women received either diclofenac (n = 25) or placebo (n = 25) suppository at the end of surgery. Subsequent postoperative pain relief was prescribed in accordance with local protocols. Observations including pain intensity were recorded at the end of surgery and at regular intervals postoperatively during the first 48 hours. The mean time to first analgesia was significantly longer in women who received diclofenac compared with those who received placebo, but the additional analgesia required was similar in both groups The authors attribute this to the efficacy of spinal morphine which meant that the overall scores for pain on mobilising was low in both groups. Although no serious atony was recorded in this study, side-effects were recorded and whilst there were no statistically significant differences between groups, for two women in the diclofenac group, the midwife recorded excessive lochia. The authors report that both these women had atonic uterus at caesarean section and before the diclofenac was given.

The numbers in these trials were small, the methods of anaesthesia and postoperative analgesia protocols differed and no systematic review has been done. While there may be some benefit from use of NSAIDs, the need to record side-effects is paramount for any future evaluations. This may be particularly important for those complications which, though rare, are peculiar to the postpartum period, and may have serious consequences for the woman and her baby.

A systematic review of trials of incisional local anaesthesia for postoperative pain relief after various procedures at abdominal surgery showed that this method was effective for up to 7 hours in inguinal herniotomy. The effect was not, however, demonstrated following hysterectomy though the studies combined still lacked the statistical power to determine whether there was an effect (Moiniche et al 1998). Caesarean section patients were not included in the review. There are therefore pitfalls in generalising findings from studies of general surgical patients.

General surgical studies suggest that postoperative pain decreases rapidly to become negligible by the fourth day after surgery (Melzack et al 1987) but this will be influenced by any complications such as wound infection. Perception of pain levels differs between the patient and their nursing staff, with nurses more commonly tending to underestimate the patient's pain (Field 1996).

In most instances, however, it is likely that by the time a woman has been discharged from hospital after a caesarean section, she will no longer require more than oral analgesia.

## Simple pain relief

In Dewan et al's 1993 study of postpartum pain, only 17% of the women treated with paracetamol for postpartum pain had good pain relief and 58% with mefenamic acid (an NSAID). Whilst some drug combinations have been compared with single agents, trials of different agents or combinations are less plentiful. The results of such reviews and studies have been pooled with a single outcome – the number of patients needed to be treated (NNT) in order that one of them will receive a 50% reduction in pain compared with a placebo (Oxford Pain Internet Site 2003). Some reservation about the robustness of the resulting league table must be retained, as the comparisons are not made within the same randomisation and conditions may differ for the drugs 'appearing to compete'. As discussed, the comparison of analgesics is sensitive to pain intensity and the results which follow relate to moderate to severe postoperative pain.

Oral NSAIDs (ibuprofen, diclofenac) are most effective. There is no evidence that giving NSAIDs rectally or by injection confers an advantage. Injected opioids need to be given at higher dose to achieve an improvement on NSAIDs; the NNT for 10 mg of IM morphine was 2.9, i.e. for every 2.9 people treated, one will get a 50% reduction in pain attributable to the drug. The NNT to get the same outcome for ibuprofen 400 mg was less and for diclofenac 50 mg was even less – approximately 2.5. For paracetamol 1000 mg alone, the NNT was almost 5. The NNT for paracetamol 650 mg + 65 mg of dextropropoxyphene was slightly lower but by adding 60 mg of codeine to the same dose of paracetamol, the NNT was reduced to just over 3. With 60 mg of codeine added to 1000 mg of paracetamol, the NNT was even slightly lower than that of diclofenac. The commonest combined tablet in the UK is paracetamol 500 mg with only 8 mg of codeine. NNTs for this combination are not quoted and there appear to be no reported trials of the efficacy of this combination. It is likely that a reduced dose of codeine has less analgesic effect but a better safety profile. However, repeated doses may be more common if pain relief is less effective, and there may be cumulative effects as a result.

A standard prescribing policy would ensure that postnatal women received appropriate pain management. Many women probably experience pain that could be alleviated, but because of failure by health professionals to acknowledge pain needs and apply consistent prescribing policies, effective care is not given. An example of a prescribing policy was presented in an audit of postoperative pain relief at home among 150 adults who attended a day surgery unit (Haynes et al 1995). Patients who underwent general surgery, ophthalmic, ENT or gynaecology procedures were asked to rate their pain as mild, moderate or severe at 24 and 72 hours and record analgesia used during this period. Around half of the patients were managed according to the hospital's prescribing policy. Of 111 returns, 29 (26%) patients reported severe pain on at least one occasion and 12 (11%) contacted their GP or were readmitted because of poor pain control. As a result, the prescribing policy was revised; procedures were ordered according to whether mild, moderate or severe pain could be expected and prescribing policy amended to take account of this. A second audit of 200 patients over a 10-week period in 1994 found that 89% of patients received pain relief according to the prescribing policy and no patients had to contact their GP for postoperative pain relief.

The following prescribing policy is based on that presented by Haynes et al (1995), and it is likely to be appropriate for postnatal women.

- Mild pain: paracetamol 1000 mg four times daily
- Moderate pain: co-codamol 1 or 2 tablets four times a day
- Severe pain: co-codamol 1 or 2 tablets four times a day plus ibuprofen 500 mg twice a day

Contraindications to NSAIDs should be taken into consideration; ibuprofen may be preferred to co-codamol for women where constipation as a possible side-effect would accentuate perineal problems. Referral to the GP will be required for analgesics stronger than co-codamol and contraindications to NSAIDs should be taken into consideration.

## SUMMARY OF THE EVIDENCE USED IN THIS GUIDELINE

- Lack of a single definition of wound infection makes evaluation of the evidence more difficult.
- Most of the data relating to complications following caesarean section are generated from retrospective case-note review and confined to the woman's time in hospital and there is little evidence of infection rates once in the community.
- Evidence from general surgery surveillance suggests that a substantial proportion of all wound infections will occur after the first week, though incidence falls after 21 days, by which time approximately 90% will have become manifest.
- There are no data on the effect of different community management factors (i.e. hygiene strategies, length and frequency of surveillance, etc.) on the occurrence or course of wound infection following section.
- There is evidence from systematic review that antibiotic prophylaxis is beneficial for caesarean section and it is recommended to all units on the basis of its efficacy in preventing endometritis. It will not eliminate wound infection completely and its influence on infections occurring later is not known.
- A strategy for the management of pain using paracetamol, co-codamol and ibuprofen may increase the number of women receiving effective pain relief.

## WHAT TO DO

### Initial assessment and general advice – All women delivered by caesarean section

- Retain a high index of suspicion for wound infection, urinary tract infection and endometritis.
- Discuss with the woman the recovery from surgery, and the potential risk of acquiring infection.
- Ask about general well-being, with particular regard to any signs of fever.
- Ask if she has received or is still taking any medication (antibiotics, analgesia). If taking antibiotics, assess the reason and stress the need to complete the course as directed. If possible, record whether antibiotic prophylaxis was used and if so which agent/s.
- Advise the woman on wound care. Tell her that wound dressings are not necessary after the first 24–48 hours if the wound is kept clean and dry.
- The woman should be encouraged to bath or shower daily. If a flannel or washcloth is used it should be freshly laundered.
- Observe the wound to establish a baseline condition. Look for new line signs of dehiscence (separation of the wound edges) and evidence of infection:
  - tenderness around the wound
  - discharge from the wound: is it purulent (i.e. pus)?
  - redness spreading from the incision line
  - localised heat or swelling around the wound site.

See below for management if dehiscence or infection suspected.

- Give advice about finding a comfortable position for infant feeding (refer to guideline on Breast Feeding Issues).
- The woman should be advised not to lift heavy objects.
- If the woman has had emergency surgery she may have a perineal wound as well. Check and if appropriate refer to guideline for Perineal Pain and Dyspareunia for perineal care.

### Pain relief

- Pain relief requirements and options should be discussed with the woman.
- If the woman has effective analgesia from the hospital, this should be continued as prescribed.
- If inadequate, or no analgesia:
  - for mild pain suggest paracetamol as required up to 4 g a day in divided doses
  - for moderate pain paracetamol may be used in combination tablets with codeine (co-codamol) according to local prescribing policy. *Repeated doses may cause adverse effects and should be avoided*

- if regular pain relief is required for moderate to severe pain, NSAIDs such as ibuprofen or diclofenac may be advised in accordance with local prescribing policy
- if the suggested medications do not fall within the remit of local policy on prescribing, appropriate referral should be made (urgent action).
- Review analgesic requirements and effectiveness at each subsequent visit.

## Wound satisfactory on initial assessment

- Inspect the wound and record findings at each postnatal visit.
- It is not possible to be entirely prescriptive about scheduling visits specifically to inspect the wound. If no signs of wound infection are apparent when the initial visit is before the fifth postnatal day, arrange to visit at least once more before day 14.
- At the last planned visit, especially if this is before 28 days, the woman should be advised that it is still possible that the wound may become infected. Encourage continued attention to hygiene and ensure that she can contact you or an appropriate health professional if she suspects a problem with the wound.

## Dehiscence suspected or evident

- If wound dehiscence is severe, emergency referral should be made. Explain to the woman and her partner that hospital admission for assessment may be required. If circumstances permit, apply sterile non-occlusive dressing.
- If bowel visible (i.e. burst abdomen) arrange immediate transfer to hospital (emergency action). Apply a wet sterile pack or pad to the wound.
- If dehiscence is superficial, treat as 'other symptoms of infection'.

## Evidence of infection detected

- Record the pulse and temperature.
- If wound is discharging or shows other signs of infection, take a swab, with a sample of pus if possible, for culture.
- In dressing the wound, it is recommended that local policy should be followed where available. If one is not available, a simple occlusive non-adherent dressing is best. If an occlusive dressing cannot be applied, the dressing should be secured with strapping to all edges to keep it secure.

- Referral should be made so that the wound can be assessed, a specialist dressing prescribed, and any additional management instituted if appropriate (urgent action).
- If sutures or clips are in situ and enough time has elapsed since surgery, remove alternate ones to allow drainage from the wound. If there is any concern regarding possible dehiscence, do not remove any clips or sutures and refer (emergency action).
- If pyrexial, advise paracetamol-based analgesia unless contraindicated. Referral should be made if temperature exceeds 38° C and fails to settle after 24 hours (emergency action).
- Look for other possible sources of infection, e.g. breast problems, respiratory tract, urinary tract, endometritis, perineal wound, and refer to the appropriate guideline.
- Reassure the woman and advise her to contact her healthcare professional if the symptoms worsen.
- Review as appropriate.

### General advice

- Take prescribed pain relief as necessary.
- If prescribed antibiotics complete the full course.
- Take care of the wound:
  - bath or shower daily
  - do not apply a dressing unless supplied by the doctor or midwife.
- Wear loose clothing, use cotton underwear.
- Take care to find a comfortable position to feed the baby.
- Do not lift heavy objects.

## SUMMARY GUIDELINE

## Caesarean section wound care and pain relief

### Initial assessment – All women delivered by caesarean section

- Ask about well-being; any signs of fever
- Determine current medication and reason for prescription
- Discuss pain relief requirements and need for vigilance re possible infection
- Assess the condition of the wound for: separation (dehiscence) of the wound edges; tenderness; discharge (type, e.g. pus/serous); redness spreading from incision line; localised heat or swelling; odour

**Emergency action is required if:**

- Evidence of infection
- Severe dehiscence

## What to do

### Wound satisfactory on initial assessment

- Inspect wound at each postnatal visit
- Retain high index of suspicion for infection
- If sutures/clips in situ, remove as per policy
- If wound appears suspect at any assessment, follow relevant sections of guideline

### Dehiscence

- If dehiscence severe, immediate referral (emergency action). Apply sterile, non-occlusive dressing if available. Use wet sterile pack or pad if bowel visible
- Explain to woman and partner that hospital admission may be required
- If dehiscence superficial, treat as other symptoms of infection

### Evidence of infection detected (pyrexia, localised pain, erythema, local oedema, excess exudate, offensive odour)

- Inspect wound and record findings
- Record pulse and temperature
- If there is exudate, take swab, apply simple occlusive dressing and refer (urgent action)
- If sutures or clips in situ, remove alternate ones if appropriate
- If pyrexial, advise paracetamol-based analgesia unless contraindicated. Refer if temperature over 38 °C or fails to settle after 24 hours (emergency action)
- Look for other possible sources of infection
- Reassure, and advise woman to contact healthcare professional if the symptoms worsen
- Review as appropriate

# References

Ausobsky JR, Evans M, Pollock AV 1985 Does mass closure of midline laparotomies stand the test of time? A randomised controlled clinical trial. Ann R Coll Surg Eng 67(3): 159-161

Beattie PG, Rings TR, Hunter MF et al 1994 Risk factors for wound infection following Caesarean section. Aust NZ J Obstet Gynaecol 34(4): 398-402

Bell FG, Fenton PA 1993 Early hospital discharge and cross infection. Lancet 342: 120

Brooten D, Roncoli M, Finkler S et al 1994 A randomized trial of early hospital discharge and home follow-up of women having cesarean birth. Obstet Gynecol 84: 832-838

Brown S, Small R, Faber B et al 2002 Early postnatal discharge from hospital for healthy mothers and term infants. Cochrane Database of Systematic Reviews, Issue 3

Bucknall TE 1983 Factors influencing wound complications: a clinical and experimental study. Ann R Coll Surg Eng 65(2): 71-77

Bush DJ, Lyons G, Macdonald R 1992 Diclofenac for analgesia after Caesarean section. Anaesthesia 47: 1075-1077

Chrintz H, Vibits H, Cordtz TO et al 1989 Need for surgical wound dressing. Br J Surg 76: 204-205

Dealey C 1994 The care of wounds. Blackwell Scientific Publications, Oxford

Dennis AR, Leeson-Payne CG, Hobbs GJ 1995 Analgesia after Caesarean section. The use of rectal diclofenac as an adjunct to spinal morphine. Anaesthesia 50: 297-299

Department of Health 1997 NHS maternity statistics, England 1989–90 to 1994–95. Statistical bulletin 1997/28. Department of Health, London

Department of Health 2005 NHS maternity statistics, England: 2003–04. Statistical bulletin 2005/10. Department of Health, London

Dewan G, Glazener C, Tunstall M 1993 Postnatal pain: a neglected area. Br J Midwif 1(2): 63-66

Donald I 1979 Practical obstetric problems, 5th edn. Pitman Press, Bath

Field L 1996 Are nurses still underestimating patients' pain post operatively? Br J Nurs 5(13): 778-784

Francome C, Savage WD, Churchill H et al 1993 Caesarean birth in Britain. Middlesex University Press, London

Hawrylyshyn PA, Bernstein P, Papsin FR 1981 Risk factors associated with infection following caesarean section. Am J Obstet Gynecol 139: 294-298

Haynes TK, Evans DE, Roberts D 1995 Pain relief after day surgery: quality improvement by audit. Journal of One-Day Surgery 4(4): 12-15

Henderson E, Love EJ 1995 Incidence of hospital-acquired infections associated with caesarean section. J Hosp Infect 29: 245-255

Hillan EM 1992 Short-term morbidity associated with caesarean delivery. Birth 19: 190-194

Hillan EM 1995 Postoperative morbidity following caesarean delivery. J Adv Nurs 22: 1035-1042

Hulton LJ, Olmsted RN, Treston-Aurand J et al 1992 Effect of postdischarge surveillance on rates of infectious complications after caesarean section. Am J Infect Control 20(4): 198-201

Leigh DA, Emmanuel FXS, Sedgwick J et al 1990 Post-operative urinary tract infection and wound infection in women undergoing Caesarean section: a comparison of two study periods in 1985 and 1987. J Hosp Infect 15: 107-116

Meers PD 1981 Infection in hospitals. BMJ Clinical Research Edition 282(6271): 1246-1981

Melzack R, Abbott FV, Zackon W et al 1987 Pain on a surgical ward: a survey of the duration and intensity of pain and the effectiveness of medication. Pain 29: 67-72

Moiniche S, Mikkelsen S, Wetterslev J et al 1998 A qualitative systematic review of incisional local anaesthesia for postoperative pain relief after abdominal operations. Br J Anaesth 81: 377-383

Moir-Bussy BR, Hutton RM, Thompson JR 1984 Wound infection after caesarean section. J Hosp Infect 5: 359-370

Morrison MJ 1992 A colour guide to the nursing management of wounds. Wolfe, London

National Institute for Health and Clinical Excellence (NICE) 2004 Caesarean section. NICE Clinical Guideline no. 13.

National Institute for Health and Clinical Excellence 2006. Postnatal care: Routine postnatal care of women and their babies. NICE Clinical Guidelines 37

Nice C, Feeney A, Godwin P et al 1996 A prospective audit of wound infection rates after caesarean section in five West Yorkshire hospitals. J Hosp Infect 33: 55-61

Oxford Pain Internet Site 2003 Available online at: www.jr2.ox.ac.uk/bandolier/booth/painpag/

Parrott T, Evans AJ, Lowes A et al 1989 Infection following caesarean section. J Hosp Infect 13: 349-354

Pirwany IR, Mahmood T 1997 Audit of infective morbidity following caesarean section at a district general hospital. Obstet Gynaecol 17(5): 439-443

Rorarius MG, Suominen P, Baer GA et al 1993 Diclofenac and ketoprofen for pain treatment after elective Caesarean section. Br J Anaesth 70(3): 293-297

Savage W, Francome C 1993 British caesarean section rates: have we reached a plateau? Br J Obstet Gynaecol 100: 493-496

Smaill F, Hofmeyr GJ 2002 Antibiotic prophylaxis for cesarean section. Cochrane Database of Systematic Reviews, Issue 3. Update Software, Oxford

Tallon RW 1996 Wound care dressings. Nurs Manage 27(10): 68-70

Thomas J, Paranjothy S 2001 Royal College of Obstetricians and Gynaecologists Clinical Effectiveness Support Unit. National Sentinel Caesarean Section Audit Report. RCOG Press, London

Thomas S 1990 Wound dressings and wound management. Pharmaceutical Press, London

Thompson JR, Hutton RM, Moir-Bussy BP 1987 Estimating the infection rate in mothers following caesarean section. J Hosp Infect 10: 138-144

Weigelt JA, Dryer D, Haley RW 1992 The necessity and efficiency of wound surveillance after discharge. Arch Surg 127(1): 77-82

Chapter **4**

# Breastfeeding issues

Women need consistent advice on breastfeeding matters. In this guideline we have made every effort to ensure that advice is consistent with two important publications: *Successful breastfeeding* (RCM 2002), recommended by the College for all midwives to read, and *Bestfeeding* (Renfrew et al 2004), an international publication for breastfeeding women, from which material has been drawn. In addition the 10 steps of the UNICEF/WHO Baby Friendly Initiative are described.

## INTRODUCTION

Breastfeeding has many health advantages for both mother and baby. Breast milk has been shown to protect babies against gastrointestinal, urinary, respiratory and middle ear infection (Howie et al 1990, Marild et al 1990, 2004), atopic disease if there is a family history of atopy (Burr et al 1989, Fewtrell 2004, Oddy et al 1999), and juvenile-onset insulin-dependent diabetes mellitus (Sadauskaite-Kuehne et al 2004). There is also evidence to indicate that breastfed babies have a reduced risk of becoming obese (Arenz et al 2004, Fewtrell 2004). Maternal benefits include reduced risk of premenopausal breast cancer and some forms of ovarian cancer (Department of Health 1994) and a possibility of protection against hip fractures in older age (Department of Health 1998). In addition, breastfeeding provides a unique maternal–infant contact and ready availability of food for the baby.

Despite robust evidence to support the benefits of breastfeeding and international initiatives to support practice (see next section), rates in the UK are among the lowest in Europe. The 2000 Infant Feeding Survey (Hamlyn et al 2002) found that only 62% of women overall in the UK initiated breastfeeding, but noted small increases in incidence across the four countries of the UK. The Infant Feeding Survey 2005 showed an overall initiation rate of 76%, with breastfeeding rates continuing to increase across all four countries, after standardising for maternal age and social class (Bolling et al 2007). Initial breastfeeding rates were 78% in England, 70% in Scotland, 67% in Wales and 63% in Northern Ireland. Although the 2005 survey showed an increase in the prevalence of breastfeeding up to 9 months in England, Wales and Northern Ireland compared with 2000, in line with previous surveys many women reverted to artificial feeding within a few weeks of birth (Bolling et al 2007, Foster et al 1997, Hamlyn et al 2002), just over half within 6 weeks of the birth in the 2005 survey (Bolling et al 2007). The recommended minimum duration of breastfeeding is at least 6 months to ensure that the infant receives the full protective benefits of breast milk (WHO 2002).

A number of recent policy initiatives support the need to increase the uptake and duration of breastfeeding, including The Priorities and Planning Framework 2003–2006 (Department of Health 2003), the National Service Framework for Children, Young People and Maternity Services (Department of Health 2004) and the NICE postnatal care guideline (NICE 2006). Evidence to support this chapter has also been drawn from a systematic review and evidence into action briefing published by NICE as part of the agency's work to inform public health (Dyson et al 2006, Renfrew et al 2005). Problems with assessing the evidence in relation to interventions to support the uptake and duration of breastfeeding include variation in timing of follow-up, lack of clarity around definitions of exclusive and mixed breast- and bottlefeeding, and retrospective study designs.

## HEALTHCARE ENVIRONMENT AND THE BABY FRIENDLY INITIATIVE

The NICE postnatal care guideline (2006) has recommended that all maternity units in England and Wales introduce a structured training programme to support breastfeeding, using the WHO/UNICEF Baby Friendly Initiative (BFI) as a minimum standard. The BFI is a global initiative which was launched in 1992 to encourage maternity units to support breastfeeding through implementation of the 10 steps described below, and was introduced into the UK in 1994. In order to achieve full accreditation as a BFI hospital, an external review has to be undertaken to assess that all 10 steps have been implemented. Full accreditation lasts for 2 years, following which reassessment of the standards is undertaken over a period of 3 days. Intervals between subsequent assessment will depend on how well standards are being maintained. Units can also apply for a certificate of commitment, which is awarded if there is a breastfeeding policy in place, an action plan to achieve BFI and commitment to implement the plan. Currently, only around 10% of babies in England are born in units which have BFI accreditation, compared with 58% of babies born in Scotland, 46% in Wales and 39% in Northern Ireland (data from BFI website accessed 28 March 2008).

The 10 steps of the BFI are as follows. All providers of maternity services should:

1. have a written breastfeeding policy that is routinely communicated to all healthcare staff
2. train all healthcare staff in the skills necessary to implement the breastfeeding policy
3. inform all pregnant mothers about the benefits and management of breastfeeding
4. help mothers initiate breastfeeding soon after birth
5. show mothers how to breastfeed and how to maintain lactation even if they are separated from their babies
6. give newborn infants no food or drink, other than breast milk, unless medically indicated
7. practise rooming-in, allowing mothers and infants to remain together 24 hours a day
8. encourage breastfeeding on demand
9. give no artificial teats or dummies to breastfeeding infants
10. foster the establishment of breastfeeding support groups and refer mothers to them on discharge from the hospital or clinic.

The effect of BFI implementation on breastfeeding rates in Scotland was recently evaluated in an observational study using an annual survey of progress towards achieving BFI status and annual breastfeeding rates (Broadfoot et al 2005). Breastfeeding statistics were collected when the Guthrie screening test was carried out at 7 days postpartum. Data were collected from maternity units which had over 50 births a year between 1995 and 2002 (n = 33), which provided data on 464,246 births. Women giving birth during this period were 28% (odds ratio (OR) 1.28, 95% confidence interval (CI) 1.24 1.31) more likely to be breastfeeding at 7 days if they gave birth in a hospital with the UK BFI award. Results were adjusted for mother's age, deprivation score, hospital size and year of birth. From 1995 breastfeeding rates increased significantly faster in hospitals with BFI status (11.39% cf 7.97%). Impact on duration was not investigated as part of this study.

A more recent study (Bartington et al 2006) aimed to examine if women were more likely to commence and continue breastfeeding if they gave birth in a BFI-accredited unit in the UK, in a cohort with a high representation of women from disadvantaged and lower socio-economic groups. Women were asked to report if they had commenced breastfeeding and were still breastfeeding at 1 month after birth. Data on 17,359 singleton babies were grouped according to maternity unit BFI participation status at the time of the birth (accredited, certificated or neither award). Women who had given birth in an accredited unit were more likely to commence breastfeeding (adjusted rate ratio (ARR) 1.10, 95% CI 1.05–1.15), but were not more likely to breastfeed at 1 month (0.96, 95% CI 0.84–1.09), after adjusting for social, demographic and obstetric characteristics. Breastfeeding uptake was also independently associated with attendance at antenatal classes (1.14, 95% CI 1.11–1.17), vaginal birth (1.05, 95% CI 1.03–1.08), having a companion at the birth (1.09, 95% CI 1.04–1.1.6) and hospital postnatal stay of longer than 24 hours (1.06, 95% CI 1.04–1.09).

Much of the other evidence to support the implementation of the BFI has come from countries outside the UK, with studies from high- and low-income countries represented. A controlled, non-randomised study undertaken in Italy (Cattaneo & Buzette 2001) reported outcomes on breastfeeding rates before and after staff training for BFI. The study was undertaken in eight hospitals (no Italian hospitals at the time had achieved BFI accreditation). Data on breastfeeding rates were collected at hospital discharge and at 3 and 6 months after the birth. Hospitals were allocated to one of two groups. Following an initial period of assessment in both groups, local facilitators in group 1 were trained following an adapted programme based on BFI, which they then cascaded to the health professionals at their unit. A second assessment phase was undertaken and the intervention replicated in group 2. A third and final period of assessment was undertaken in both groups 5 months after training was completed. Data collection tools included a self-assessment tool to ascertain the extent of implementation of each of the 10 BFI steps, assessment of usual hospital practice at each point in time, a self-administered questionnaire for health professionals, interviews with mothers at discharge and a telephone interview at 3 and 6 months. All hospitals showed an improvement in compliance with each of the 10 steps. Health-care professionals' knowledge of breastfeeding improved, although response rates from both groups were low. Following training there was a significant increase in mothers reporting exclusive breastfeeding at discharge, full breastfeeding at 3 months, and any breastfeeding at 6 months, although the proportion of women breastfeeding at these points in time were below recommended rates, and could have reflected a lack of support for breastfeeding in the community.

A cluster randomised controlled trial (RCT) conducted in the Republic of Belarus (PROBIT study) assessed the effects of breastfeeding promotion on breastfeeding duration and exclusivity and rates of infant respiratory and gastrointestinal infection and atopic eczema during a 1-year follow-up (Kramer et al 2001). Thirty one maternity hospitals and polyclinics were randomly assigned to receive an intervention based on the BFI (n = 16) or current care (n = 15) of usual infant practices and policies. Over 17,000 mother–infant dyads were recruited, 16,491 of whom completed the 12 months of follow-up. There was a significant increase in the duration of breastfeeding to 12 months, increased exclusive breastfeeding to 6 months, and a significant reduction in the numbers of infants who had gastrointestinal tract infections and atopic eczema, but no improvement in respiratory outcomes.

DiGirolamo and colleagues (2001) carried out a longitudinal cohort study in the USA to assess the impact of the type and number of BFI practices experienced by mothers on breastfeeding outcomes. Data were collected from the 1993–94 *Infant feeding practices survey*, a longitudinal survey of pregnant and new mothers up to 12 months after their delivery from across the USA, conducted by the United States Food and Drug Administration. The main outcome measure was breastfeeding cessation within 6 weeks of giving birth.

Of 2610 women deemed eligible for the study, 1737 (67%) returned the antenatal and subsequent postnatal questionnaires. There were imbalances in the characteristics of responders who were more likely to be white, over 30 years of age, married and to have higher income levels and educational achievements. The focus of the study was the 1085 women who reported an intention to breastfeed for more than 2 months after their delivery. The impact of five of the 10 BFI steps was assessed: breastfeeding initiation within 1 hour of the birth; feeding only breast milk; rooming-in; breastfeeding on demand; no use of dummies. Seventeen percent of women had given up breastfeeding within 6 weeks. Only 7% of the mothers had experienced all five steps, the strongest risk factors for early cessation being late commencement of a first breastfeed and supplementation of the infant. When compared to women who experienced all five steps, mothers who experienced none were eight times more likely to stop breastfeeding within 6 weeks (OR 7.7, 95% CI 2.3–25.8).

Philipp et al (2001) compared breastfeeding initiation rates at Boston Medical Center, USA, prior to (1995), during (1998) and after (1999) the BFI was implemented. Two hundred complete medical records randomly selected by computer were reviewed for each of the 3 years. Data collected from the records enabled infants to be categorised into four groups: exclusively breastfed; mostly breast milk; mostly formula; and exclusively formula. The maternal and infant demographics for all 3 years were comparable. Full implementation of the 10 steps leading to BFI accreditation resulted in significant increases in breastfeeding initiation rates from 58% in 1995 to 77.5% in 1998 to 86.5% in 1999 (p<0.001), leading the authors to conclude that full implementation of the BFI was an effective strategy to increase breastfeeding initiation rates in the US hospital setting.

The Department of Health has estimated that the NHS could save £35 million each year in the treatment of babies with gastroenteritis alone, if all babies were breastfed, representing a saving of £300,000 for the average health district (Department of Health 1995), a saving which is likely to be significantly higher at today's costs. The NICE postnatal care guideline included the outcome of an economic model of the likely effects of universal implementation of the BFI in English and Welsh hospitals, over a 15-year period based on breastfeeding rates, and association between breastfeeding and disease occurrence (NICE 2006). This involved estimating the likely cost of universal (and ongoing) accreditation and the effect of increased breastfeeding initiation on infant health outcomes, which included gaster-oenteritis, otitis media, asthma and necrotising enterocolitis. The model showed that over a 15-year period, cost savings following implementation would outweigh the net costs of introduction of the BFI into each unit, breaking even after 6 years. An increase in breastfeeding rates attributable to the BFI of 10% over 15 years could bring an average annual saving of £8.27 million, the major part of the savings accruing from the impact of an increase in breastfeeding uptake on reductions in infant gastroenteritis. Further evidence is required of savings which would accrue from an increased duration of breastfeeding.

## SUCCESSFUL BREASTFEEDING

Breastfeeding support should be seen as an integral part of the role of the midwife providing postnatal care, and all healthcare professionals who have contact with postnatal women should have the appropriate competencies to support women to breastfeed (NICE 2006). The Royal College of Midwives (RCM) publication *Successful breastfeeding* (2002), which aimed to make breastfeeding advice offered by midwives consistent and evidence based, stressed that this advice should be given equal priority with other aspects of care.

A Cochrane systematic review of interventions to promote the initiation of breastfeeding included data from seven trials involving 1388 women (Dyson et al 2005). A meta-analysis based on five trials involving 582 women on low incomes in the USA showed that breastfeeding education had a significant effect on increasing initiation rates compared to routine care (relative risk (RR) 1.53, 95% CI 1.25–1.88). However, the extent to which this effect would be found based on populations from other countries would have to be considered.

The impact of placing a baby on his/her mother's chest as soon as possible after birth or within the first 24 hours of the birth (termed 'skin-to-skin contact') has been assessed in relation to breastfeeding uptake and duration. A Cochrane review by Anderson et al (2003) included 17 RCTs which provided data on 806 mother–infant dyads. The methodological quality of most of the studies was poor and intervention characteristics, such as duration of skin-to-skin contact, varied greatly across the studies. Data were obtained from diverse populations from a range of countries. Fifteen studies included only women who had given birth vaginally and all but one study included only healthy, full-term babies. More skin-to-skin dyads were still breast-feeding 1–3 months (30–90 days) post birth (OR 2.15, 95% CI 1.10–4.22). The reviewers concluded that early skin-to-skin contact appeared to have some clinical benefit especially regarding breastfeeding outcomes and infant crying and had no apparent short- or long-term negative effects. Study data showed that most of the infants suckled during the skin-to-skin intervention, which may be a critical component of this intervention with regard to long-term breastfeeding success. Although further research is required, it appears women and their infants should not be separated following the birth without an unavoidable medical reason.

A recent RCT undertaken in the north of England, and not included in the above review, also examined the effects of skin-to-skin care on breastfeeding outcomes (Carfoot et al 2005). Two hundred and four women and their infants were randomised to routine care (n = 102) or immediate skin-to-skin care (n = 102). The infants in the usual care group were dried and wrapped in a towel before being handed to their mother or father. In the skin-to-skin group infants were placed prone against their mother's skin and between her breasts as soon as possible after birth. The primary outcome was success of the first breastfeed, as assessed using the Infant Breast Feeding Assessment Tool (IBFAT). Secondary outcomes included breastfeeding at 4 months and infant body temperature at 1 hour after the birth. There were no statistically significant differences between the two groups on successful first feed or breastfeeding at 4 months, although a higher proportion of babies in the skin-to-skin group had a successful first feed (91% cf 83%) and were partially or exclusively breastfeeding at 4 months (43% cf 40%). The mean infant temperature at 1 hour after birth was also higher in the skin-to-skin group, which was statistically significant (95% CI 0.03–0.28, p = 0.02), although this difference was not considered to be clinically significant. Women who had skin-to-skin contact enjoyed the experience, and most reported they would choose to have skin-to-skin care in the future.

Almost all women who decide to breastfeed will have commenced this whilst in hospital, but most will now be discharged prior to the establishment of lactation, so that midwives in the community have an even greater role to play in breastfeeding advice. Not all babies will be ready to feed within the same time period. Babies have been shown to display a wide range of feeding behaviour following a spontaneous delivery (Henschel & Inch 1996, Widstrom et al 1990).

Interventions during labour may also impact on commencement and early cessation of breastfeeding, although much of the evidence to date comes from small studies, few of which were prospective and which have produced inconclusive results. Data from a UK-wide survey of breastfeeding practices at 6 weeks postpartum found that a longer time to first feed was associated with obstetric intervention, such as induction, caesarean section and the use of pethidine during labour (Rajan 1994). A small study by Ransjö-Arvidson et al (2001) examined the impact of maternal analgesia for labour pain relief on infant behaviour. Pre-feeding infant behaviour during the first 2 hours of life was the focus of the study. A convenience sample of 28 infants whose mothers had uncomplicated pregnancies were videoed to observe for pre-feeding gestures including movement of eyes, hands and mouth, touching the nipple before suckling, rooting and licking movements. Women were grouped according to type of labour analgesia. One group had received mepivacaine via a pudendal block (n = 6), a second group had received pethidine or bupivacaine (n = 12), and a third group received no analgesia during labour (n = 10). A significantly lower proportion of babies whose mothers had received any medication touched the nipple with their hands before suckling (p<0.01), made licking movements (p<0.01) and fed (p<0.01). Small numbers limit the generalisability of the findings.

Volmanen et al (2004), in a qualitative study from Lapland, contacted 164 women to ask about problems with breastfeeding, and mixed breast and formula feeding, a median of 2.4 years after delivery. Ninety nine women returned completed questionnaires. Fifty six of these women received an epidural during labour. Although the study was limited by size and potential recall bias, those who had epidural analgesia in labour reported a higher incidence of partial breastfeeding or formula feeding (67% vs 29%; p = 0.003). The researchers speculated that infants affected by bupivacaine crossing the placental barrier (via epidural) might be less capable of stimulating lactation during the neonatal period but these findings should be treated with caution given the study limitations.

In a small well-designed cohort study, Radzyminski (2003) looked at the effect of ultra low-dose epidural analgesia on breastfeeding among 56 mother–infant dyads. Twenty eight women had epidural analgesia, with pain relief provided by low–dose fentanyl and bupivacaine, and 28 did not use any analgesia. Several methods of evaluation were employed to assess drug effects on infant feeding up to 24 hours post delivery, including a preterm infant breastfeeding behaviour scale and a neurobehaviour scale. No significant difference was demonstrated between breastfeeding behaviours of babies born to mothers who had an epidural and those who had no method of analgesia.

A prospective study from France, which also included small numbers, examined predictive factors associated with cessation of breastfeeding whilst on the postnatal ward and up to 4 months after the birth among women who gave birth in what the researchers referred to as a 'high-tech' maternity unit (the definition of this was not given) (Lathouwer et al 2004). Breastfeeding status was ascertained on the day of hospital discharge and at 1, 2, 3 and 4 months after birth. Data were collected on 115 women who gave birth during the first 2 months of 2002 and commenced breastfeeding (only 57% of 203 women who gave birth during the study period). At the time of hospital discharge which took place 4 days after the birth, six of the 115 (5.2%) women had given up breastfeeding. During these 4 days, 61% of breastfed infants received at least one supplementary feed with artificial baby milk. Cessation of breastfeeding occurred rapidly following discharge, particularly after 3 months. Of the 109 (95%) women still breastfeeding (which included exclusive and combined breast and artificial milk) on the day of discharge from hospital, 78% were still breastfeeding at 1 month, 66% at 2 months, 44% at 3 months and 17% at 4 months. When data for 'currently exclusively breastfeeding' were separated, only 69% were exclusively breastfeeding at 1 month, 47% at 2 months, 17% at 3 months and 6% at 4 months. The only factor associated with early cessation of breastfeeding during the inpatient period was defined as 'lack of experience' in multiparous women who decided to breastfeed for the first time (OR 35.33). There were no differences in breastfeeding outcomes by mode of delivery. The small numbers and absence of data on other obstetric, anaesthetic, demographic or maternal characteristics or levels of breastfeeding support during the postnatal period suggest that the results should be interpreted with caution.

A recent prospective cohort study from Australia examined the impact of epidural analgesia during labour on breastfeeding during the first postnatal week and breastfeeding cessation up to the first 24 weeks after the birth (Torvaldsen et al 2006). The study was undertaken in the Australian Capital Territory in 1997. The epidural solution in use at the time was bupivacaine 0.16% with fentanyl 3.3 µg/ml, administered as patient-controlled analgesia. One thousand two hundred and eighty women aged 16 years and over who had given birth to a single live infant were asked to complete questionnaires at 1, 8, 16 and 24 weeks after giving birth. Data were available on 1260 women, 416 (33%) of whom had epidurals. Infant feed data were categorised as either fully breastfeeding, partially breastfeeding or not breastfeeding at all. Following the first survey point, women who had stopped breastfeeding since the previous survey were asked when they stopped. Labour analgesia and mode of birth were associated with partial breastfeeding and problems with breastfeeding in the first postpartum week, a statistically significant finding (p<0.0001). Partial breastfeeding in the first week was associated with three intrapartum factors: use of intrapartum analgesia (p<0.0001), type of birth (p<0.0001) and onset of labour (p = 0.0003). Parity was also significant (p = 0.0006). After adjusting for parity, only epidurals and general anaesthetic were significantly associated with increased risk of partial breastfeeding in the first week; however, when analyses were restricted only to women who had vaginal births, this association was weaker and, after adjusting for parity, the strength of association between epidurals and partial breastfeeding was no longer statistically significant.

Breastfeeding difficulties in the first week after birth were associated with epidural analgesia, after adjusting for parity (OR 2.04, 95% CI 1.39–3.00), an association which remained significant when analyses were restricted to women who had vaginal births (OR 1.75, 95% CI 1.13–2.70). Breastfeeding cessation in the first 24 weeks was associated with analgesia, maternal age and level of education (p < 0.0001). Women who had received an epidural analgesia were more likely to stop breastfeeding than women who had used non-pharmacological methods of pain relief (adjusted hazard ratio 2.02, 95% CI 1.53–2.67). The fact that none of the intrapartum factors was associated with not breastfeeding at all highlights that breastfeeding uptake is more likely to be related to social factors.

The 2000 *Infant feeding survey* (Hamlyn et al 2002) found that 12% of women who commenced breastfeeding gave up whilst still on the postnatal ward. It also found that being given artificial milk whilst in hospital was associated with stopping breastfeeding within the first 2 weeks; 40% of mothers whose babies had been given a bottle in hospital stopped breastfeeding, compared with 13% of women whose babies had not been given a bottle (Hamlyn et al 2002). In the 2005 survey, a third of breastfed babies had received additional feeds of formula, water or glucose whilst in hospital (Bolling et al 2007).

Renfrew et al (2005), in a systematic review of the effectiveness of public health interventions to promote the duration of breastfeeding, reviewed five RCTs and two non-RCTs and concluded that supplements in the neonatal period should be given only when there are sound medical indications, which supports the WHO/UNICEF recommendation included in the BFI 10 steps. If supplements are given for medical reasons or mothers' choice the duration of breastfeeding is less likely to be affected if only a small number of supplements are given in the first 5 days. The reasons for introducing supplementation were examined in an ethnographic study undertaken at one maternity unit in England to explore women's and healthcare professionals' beliefs, expectations and experiences in relation to supplementation of breastfeeding in the postnatal ward and neonatal unit (Cloherty et al 2004). Mothers who planned to breastfeed but were supplementing their babies with formula feed or expressed breast milk were invited to take part. One of the themes generated related to the conflict of the midwives' role to support breastfeeding with their desire to protect women from tiredness or distress, a theme confirmed by the mothers' accounts of how they felt. In some cases, the midwives suggested supplementation whilst in other cases it was requested by the mother. The importance of healthcare professionals being aware of other solutions to assist a breastfeeding mother who is tired and distressed should clearly be a priority (see Chapter 8 on Fatigue).

The length of stay on the postnatal ward has reduced considerably in the UK as a consequence of a number of drivers, including cost containment (Renfrew et al 2005). The impact of reduced inpatient care on maternal and infant health outcomes and feeding practices has been considered in several studies, although changes in service provision have tended to only include breastfeeding as a secondary outcome. The effect on the duration of breastfeeding was evaluated by Brown & Lumley (1997), in a study from Australia. The researchers assessed the impact of early discharge on maternal health outcomes, including duration of breastfeeding in women who gave birth 6–7 months previously at hospitals in Victoria. At 6 weeks, 3 months and 6 months small, non-significant differences were observed in the pattern of infant feeding of women who were discharged within 48 hours and those who stayed 5 or more days after birth. Women who left hospital on day 3 or 4 had significantly lower rates of breastfeeding at 6 weeks (OR 0.58, 95% CI 0.4–0.8), 3 months (OR 0.6, 95% CI 0.5–0.8) and 6 months (OR 0.74, 95% CI 0.6–0.96).

A Cochrane review by Brown and colleagues (2002) considered the safety, impact and effectiveness of a policy of early postnatal discharge for healthy women and their term babies, where 'early discharge' referred to discharge that was earlier than standard care in the setting in which the intervention was implemented. The pooled estimate from six trials which reported data on partial or exclusive breastfeeding at 1 or 2 months postpartum suggested no significant difference between women who had early hospital discharge and the control group who received standard care (pooled RR 0.96, 95% CI 0.78–01.18). However, there was significant heterogeneity between the trials included in this analysis (for example, cultural differences in duration of breastfeeding, and different measures used to assess breastfeeding).

A large longitudinal cohort study from Sweden (Waldenström & Aarts 2004) investigated the duration of breastfeeding and number of breastfeeding problems, with a focus on association with the length of postpartum stay. Women attending for their first antenatal clinic appointment were recruited from all clinics in Sweden over 3 weeks evenly spread over a 1-year period. Data on any breastfeeding were collected by postal questionnaire at 2 months and 1 year post delivery. Data on 2709 women (82% of the 3293 who originally agreed to participate) who completed questions on length of stay included in the 2-month questionnaire were presented in this paper. Women were divided into six groups according to length of postnatal stay (day 1 <24 h to day 6 ≥120 h). A number of statistical tests were undertaken to examine the effect of length of stay and potential confounding factors on duration of breastfeeding. Kaplan Meier analysis showed the unadjusted median duration of any breastfeeding was 7 months in women discharged from the postnatal ward on day 1 post delivery and 8 months in women discharged on any of the following days, a non-significant difference (p = 0.66). The difference remained non-significant after adjustment for interrelated maternal characteristics. The authors concluded that maternal characteristics and their experience of their first breastfeed may be more important predictors of breastfeeding duration than length of inpatient care.

Observational studies that have investigated infant feeding have consistently reported that younger women, those from lower socio-economic groups and of younger age when leaving full-time education are less likely to breastfeed (Bick et al 1998, Hally et al 1984). Since most studies have employed large-scale quantitative techniques, subtle social and cultural influences that could affect decisions about infant feeding may not have been identified. A qualitative study of 21 women, which sought to improve understanding of how primiparae belonging to lower income groups had decided to feed their infants, suggested that breastfeeding is a skill which needs to be learnt, particularly by women with little exposure to other breastfeeding women (Hoddinott & Pill 1999). These authors suggest that women may benefit from an antenatal apprenticeship with a known breast-feeding mother. Low rates of breastfeeding over the past two decades mean that many women may not have access within their social network to an effective role model.

A cluster RCT in Mexico City assessed the effects of two different models of home-based peer counselling on the proportion of women exclusively breastfeeding at 3 months (Morrow et al 1999). One hundred and thirty women participated: 44 received six visits, two in pregnancy and at 2, 4 and 8 weeks postpartum; 52 received one visit in pregnancy and two visits at 1 and 2 weeks postpartum; and 34 received usual care (controls). The home visits were made by peer counsellors recruited from within the same community as the women, who had been trained by the La Leche League. Antenatal visits focused on the benefits of exclusive breastfeeding, the importance of positioning, and discussion of solutions to common breast-feeding problems. Postnatal visits focused on maternal concerns, information and social support. Both intervention groups were found to be significantly more likely to be exclusively breastfeeding at 3 months than the controls, which was practised by 28 (67%) of the six-visit group, 25 (50%) of the three-visit group and four (12%) of the control group. These findings were not related to any of the sociodemographic, delivery or health factors examined. However, further research is necessary in other communities since findings may not be applicable across cultures.

Additional support during the postnatal period for women who are breastfeeding does appear to be effective. Renfrew et al (2005) found high-quality evidence from two studies of the benefit of health professional and peer support on both exclusive and any breastfeeding among women from relatively advantaged communities, and evidence from another two studies of a lesser quality, both of which were targeted at African-American women from disadvantaged backgrounds, that support can be effective for any breastfeeding. Postnatal interventions which did not include specific additional breastfeeding support had no beneficial impact, and no evidence was found of effective interventions to support exclusive breastfeeding among disadvantaged women.

Tools to enable women and healthcare professionals to assess progress with breastfeeding have also been evaluated. Hamelin & McLennan (2000), in a study from Canada, assessed the relationship between the use of the LATCH Breastfeeding Charting System by nursing staff during postpartum hospitalisation and breastfeeding outcomes. A post-test control group design with non-random groups collected data from a convenience sample of 180 breastfeeding women who gave birth in an urban perinatal centre. Ninety women received the LATCH tool intervention, which assigned a numerical score of 0, 1 or 2 to five key components of breastfeeding. Six-week postpartum telephone interviews demonstrated no significant differences in breast-feeding outcomes between the two groups in exclusive breastfeeding, although women in the post-test group reported increased confidence in their assessment of infant breastfeeding and when to ask for help with breastfeeding problems. The use of the tool did not reduce the incidence of early breastfeeding problems, particularly women's concerns about per-ceived insufficient breast milk, which was reported by a similar proportion in both groups (50% cf 46%).

Two studies which had considered the effectiveness of breastfeeding self-assessment tools were included in the review by Renfrew et al (2005). A study by Pollard (1998) conducted in the USA among women of different socio-economic groups evaluated the effectiveness of a breastfeeding self-monitoring daily log book in addition to a breastfeeding education session, including a video and question and answer session. A significant increase in mean duration of breastfeeding was demonstrated amongst women who adhered to the protocol, although these were likely to be married women, from higher socio-economic groups. They breastfed their infants for three times longer than women who were single who had been uncertain about breastfeeding and had not completed self-monitoring forms. The second study (Loh et al 1997) evaluated use of a simple fact sheet covering eight positive aspects of breastfeeding during the late antenatal period adminis-tered by medical students to women attending one antenatal clinic who were randomised to an intervention group and a control group. This resulted in a 38% increase in breastfeeding rates at hospital discharge in the intervention group and a similar increase in breastfeeding rates 4 weeks after the birth but this was not statistically significant, probably due to small numbers in the trial; 193 women were recruited across the two trial arms.

Renfrew and colleagues (2005) concluded that use of education interven-tions delivered through the use of a self-assessment tool appears to have the potential to increase the duration of breastfeeding among some groups of women, but care would be required to ensure tools were tailored for the intended population. With respect to the second study, further research was required based on larger numbers, with adequate sample size, and con-sideration given to issues such as method of randomisation and the most appropriate healthcare professional to deliver such an intervention. The review did not find any evidence of effectiveness of the use of written mate-rials alone to support breastfeeding (Renfrew et al 2005).

A high proportion of early breastfeeding problems may be due to incor-rect positioning of the baby on the breast. Renfrew et al (2005) considered the evidence from one Australian RCT (n = 75), in which the intervention comprised a group educational session on positioning and attachment of the baby at the breast for primiparous women on low incomes, who stated their intention to breastfeed (Duffy et al 1997). Study outcomes showed an increased duration of exclusive breastfeeding at 6 weeks postpartum, Renfrew and colleagues (2005) concluding that the trial was of high quality which should support the widespread replication of this intervention amongst similar population groups in the UK.

Despite efforts to ensure that appropriate advice and support are given, there are frequent complaints from mothers of inconsistent advice from healthcare professionals about breastfeeding (RCM 2002). It is essential that professionals who have contact with breastfeeding women are regularly updated on breastfeeding matters.

## BREASTFEEDING PROBLEMS

It is likely that almost all postnatal breastfeeding problems can be prevented if the baby is able to feed effectively and efficiently from the beginning (Inch & Fisher 1999). This does not always occur, however, so in addition to having knowledge about how to achieve effective, pain-free breastfeeding, all midwives need to know how to manage breastfeeding problems.

### Painful nipples

Painful nipples were reported by women in the Infant Feeding Survey 2005 as one of the main reasons for discontinuing breastfeeding (Bolling et al 2007), with a quarter of women who stopped breastfeeding within the first week of giving birth citing this as the reason. Trauma can occur if appropriate positioning and attachment on the breast have not been adopted, as the strong suction exerted by the baby will soon damage the nipple. Unless a baby is correctly positioned and attached to feed, there will be little or no benefit from offering other advice, support and help.

Renfrew et al (2005) reviewed four studies relevant to *preventing* painful nipples, one which considered the role of positioning education and three which considered the use of topical applications to the nipple. They concluded that teaching interventions needed to be assessed in larger studies and there was no convincing evidence that use of topical applications would prevent nipple pain. The reviewers also identified three studies which had assessed outcomes following topical applications to *treat* painful nipples, which included hydrogel dressings, tea bags, lanolin and air drying (Renfrew et al 2005), and likewise concluded that none of the interventions assessed was effective. An earlier review by Renfrew et al (2000) included evidence from three studies of nipple shields, which found no beneficial effect from their use on breastfeeding duration, milk transfer or milk volume.

It is possible that use of topical agents could detract from support to enable the women to commence and continue to experience painless breastfeeding through correct positioning and attachment. More information is required to establish why many women continue to experience sore nipples, despite being informed of appropriate feeding techniques.

### Engorgement

Engorgement results from venous congestion due to the increased blood supply to the breasts when the milk comes in. The volume of milk, if not removed as it is formed, will exceed the capacity of the alveoli to store it.

Seepage of milk into the surrounding tissues will cause a reaction (because milk is a foreign protein) but not infection; women may experience pyrexia and tachycardia and breasts become red, tense, tender and full. Unrestricted early feeding and appropriate attachment of the baby at the breast are the most effective measures to prevent engorgement.

Renfrew and colleagues (2005) identified three small trials which assessed interventions to treat engorgement, all of which tested the effectiveness of the application of cabbage leaves to the engorged breast. Two trials found some evidence of effectiveness following the application of cabbage leaves, but no advantage in using chilled as opposed to room temperature leaves, and that women preferred to use cabbage leaves than gel pads. Evidence from larger trials is now required.

## Insufficient milk

A perceived inadequate supply of breast milk was the most common reason for cessation of breastfeeding between 1 week and 4 months after the birth in the Infant Feeding Survey 2005 (Bolling et al 2007). Women may not be aware of the physiological processes of breastfeeding and as a consequence, lack confidence in their ability to feed their infants. Advice from health professionals that might have helped women to overcome this may not have been offered (Henschel & Inch 1996). It is difficult to obtain objective evidence of insufficient milk (Enkin et al 2000). However, a very small minority of women may genuinely be unable to lactate adequately (Neifert et al 1986) and there is evidence from a prospective cohort study of 630 women of an association between postpartum anaemia in the immediate postnatal period and insufficient milk (Henley et al 1995). There are no randomised controlled trials of treatments for perceived or genuine milk insufficiency and research into this is urgently required.

## Thrush

Painful nipples or acute breast pain may result from candidiasis infection (thrush). This can affect the nipples and areola and without treatment may spread to the rest of the breast or to both breasts; the infant might also have oral or perianal thrush. Thrush may occur when a mother has experienced no problems with breastfeeding, but has pain after a feed which can be severe and prolonged. The nipple and areola become red and inflamed and sensitive to touch. Women who have received antibiotics (for example, prophylactic antibiotics for caesarean section or antibiotic treatment for mastitis) will be more at risk of developing thrush (Amir 1991). Treatment from the GP is required and some candida organisms may be resistant to antifungal preparations. Nystatin suspension is usually prescribed for the baby and Canestan cream for the mother, but this needs to be washed off the breast prior to each feed. Expert opinion suggests that myconazel gel, which is an oral preparation available for use by babies, could be applied to the breast to treat the mother without the necessity of removal and, if applied before and after the feed, would also treat the baby. If local treatment fails, systemic treatment may be required, but evidence of the effectiveness of this is needed (Lawrence 1994).

## Blocked milk duct

There is sometimes no obvious cause of a blocked duct, but it can occur as a result of incomplete emptying of a lobe due to ineffective positioning or attachment of the baby to feed, or pressure placed on the breast, for example from a badly fitting bra. As a result of the obstruction, the flow of milk builds up to form a hard lump, which the woman may report as being tender. In the absence of trial evidence, 'best practice' recommends that the mother be shown how to position and attach the baby to feed, to ensure all areas of the breast are effectively drained, and how to gently 'massage' the lump towards the nipple when the baby is feeding to aid the flow of milk (Henschel & Inch 1996).

## Inverted or non-protractile nipples

Inverted or non-protractile nipples occur in about 7–10% of women (Alexander et al 1992), and women who have these may experience difficulties attaching their babies to the breast. It is the protractility of the surrounding tissue, rather than the shape of the nipple, that will determine a baby's ability to make an effective 'teat' from the breast (RCM 2002).

Antenatal treatments for inverted or non-protractile nipples have included the use of breast shells (Woolwich shells), Hoffman's exercises, surgery and a recently developed device called a 'Niplette'. Two randomised controlled trials examined Hoffman's exercises alone, breast shells alone, both breast shells and Hoffman's exercises, and no treatment (Alexander et al 1992, MAIN Trial Collaborative Group 1994). Both trials found no increase in breastfeeding duration in women who used either of the treatments separately, or both in combination. That flat or inverted nipples are not a contraindication to breastfeeding was shown in the MAIN trial, in which 45% of women with inverted or non-protractile nipples breastfed for at least 6 weeks, and women should be reassured by these findings (MAIN Collaborative Group 1994). The 'Niplette' is a nipple mould placed over the nipple and areola. A syringe is used to apply suction to the device to draw out the nipple. There is currently only one paper that has described the use of this device in which the case histories of 14 women who went on to breastfeed following use of the 'Niplette' are reported (McGeorge 1994), but the device has not been subjected to clinical evaluation.

## Mastitis

Mastitis is an inflammatory reaction to pressure placed on the breast, for example from restrictive clothing or ineffective emptying of the breast, or if a mother has missed feeds. It can be infective or non-infective, is usually painful and in most cases affects one breast. The prevalence of mastitis among breastfeeding women in the UK is unknown, but prospective studies undertaken in other countries have reported variation in incidence and prevalence. Differences may be due to case definitions, selection bias and characteristics of the study population.

A prevalence of 20% was reported in an Australian prospective cohort study, with most cases occurring within 7 weeks of delivery (Kinlay et al 1998). A prospective cohort study which followed 946 breastfeeding women who had given birth in Michigan and Nebraska during 1994–98 for 3 months after the birth, or until they stopped breastfeeding, aimed to describe the incidence of mastitis, treatment and associations with maternal and breastfeeding characteristics (Foxman et al 2002). Telephone interviews with the women were conducted at 3, 6, 9 and 12 weeks; 9.5% of women reported clinician-diagnosed lactation mastitis at least once during the first 12 weeks, 64% of these cases being diagnosed over the phone. Logistic regression analyses found history of mastitis with a previous child (OR 4.0, 95% CI 2.64–6.11), nipple problems in the same week as mastitis (OR 3.4, 95% CI 2.04–5.51), using an antifungal nipple cream in the same 3-week interval as mastitis (OR 3.4, 95% CI 1.37–8.54) and among women with no prior mastitis history, using a manual breast pump (OR 3.3, 95% CI 1.92–5.62) strongly predicted mastitis.

The incidence of mastitis and breast abscess among breastfeeding women was recently investigated in an Australian study based on data combined from two studies (an RCT and a survey) to provide a cohort of women (Amir et al 2004). Primiparous women who had given birth at two hospitals on one site were recruited (n = 1311), 1193 (91%) of whom participated in a structured telephone interview at 6 months after the birth which included questions about breastfeeding problems. One hundred and seventy one women were treated with antibiotics for at least one episode of mastitis, 14.5% overall.

As a result of the difficulties in milk flow, milk collects in the alveoli, increasing the pressure. The resulting distension may be felt as a lump or lumpiness in the breast tissue. Even without infection, a substantial proportion of women may complain of flu-like symptoms. In an earlier review, Renfrew et al (2000) identified one RCT which examined three forms of mastitis, based on leucocyte count and quantitative bacterial cultivation: milk stasis, non-infective mastitis and infective mastitis. All forms improved with regular breast draining, suggesting that breastfeeding should continue with support to encourage effective drainage from the breast. If the pain and redness of mastitis do not resolve within a few hours of either altering position to ensure effective feeding from the inflamed part of the breast or expressing breast milk to resolve the symptom, the woman must be urgently referred for potential antibiotic therapy, because of the risk of an abscess developing. In the US study described above (Foxman et al 2002), 86% of the women with mastitis were prescribed antibiotics. An observational study from nearly 40 years ago, of 53 women with a total of 71 episodes of mastitis, found that if treatment was delayed by 24 hours, women were more likely to develop an abscess (Deveraux 1969).

## Breast abscess

There have been few population-based studies of breast abscesses associated with lactation, information tending to come from individual case presentations. Five of the 1193 women in the population study reported above by Amir and colleagues (2004) developed a breast abscess (0.4%), all of whom had received antibiotics prior to abscess development. Standard treatment previously consisted of incision and drainage of the abscess as an inpatient, and regular monitoring of postoperative recovery. Dixon (1988) conducted a small study to determine if breast abscesses could be treated without an operation or readmission to hospital. Six breastfeeding women who developed a breast abscess within 3–6 weeks of delivery and had received antibiotics for 48 hours were included. Initially, pus was drained from the abscess using a 19 gauge syringe and needle, followed by a 7-day course of antibiotics. Aspiration was performed three times weekly until no further pus was drained. The women were reviewed 3 weeks after the final aspiration, by which time no symptoms of infection were present. Aspiration was recommended as first-line treatment.

O'Hara et al (1996) carried out a retrospective review of the policy at Hull Royal Infirmary for the treatment of suspected breast abscess (ultrasound scan, aspiration of pus, antibiotics and repeat aspiration if necessary). Over a 2-year period, 53 patients were admitted to hospital with a suspected breast abscess; 22 were aspirated, of which 19 resolved and three required subsequent incision and drainage. Eight patients underwent primary incision and drainage, one of whom required a second drainage. The abscess discharged spontaneously in five women. The remaining 18 patients had inflammation but no focal pus, which settled with antibiotic treatment in all but two. The authors confirmed that aspiration combined with ultrasound imaging was an effective alternative to incision and drainage.

Eryilmaz and colleagues (2005), in a study from Turkey, compared outcomes following incision and drainage or needle aspiration for the treatment of breast abscess in lactating women. Over a 3-year period, women were randomised to incision and drainage (n = 23) or needle aspiration (n = 22). A range of data were collated, including the woman's age and parity, the location of the abscess, if the nipples were cracked and diameter of the abscess. In the incision and drainage group, all women were treated successfully, but one woman had recurrence of symptoms and 16 women (70%) were dissatisfied with the cosmetic outcome. In the needle aspiration group, three women were treated with a single aspiration, and 10 (45%) with multiple aspirations, although nine women did not heal appropriately and subsequently required incision and drainage in addition. Risk factors for failure in the needle aspiration group were abscesses larger than 5 cm in diameter, unusually large volumes of aspirated pus and delay in treatment. Based on their data, the researchers concluded that for abscesses smaller than 5 cm, repeated aspirations could be performed with good cosmetic outcomes, and that incision and drainage should be used for larger abscesses.

# WOMEN WHO REQUIRE ADDITIONAL BREASTFEEDING SUPPORT

## Women who have a multiple birth

The advantages of breastfeeding for multiple birth infants are likely to be greater, since more of these infants will be premature and at greater risk of morbidity. Women who have a multiple pregnancy will require additional midwifery support and advice to ensure effective breastfeeding. It is very important to reassure women that the 'supply and demand' physiology of lactation means that they will be able to provide sufficient milk for their babies, even triplets. The evidence already referred to, on support and interventions to assist the establishment of successful breastfeeding, is applicable to multiple births. However, expert advice suggests that women may benefit from adopting a feeding routine, rather than relying on demand feeding, as this may make it easier to cope with the increased workload of looking after more than one baby. Further advice on breastfeeding multiples should be sought from the Multiple Births Association and the Twins and Multiple Births Association.

## Women who wish to combine breastfeeding and employment

Between 1985 and 1990, there was an increase in the number of women who gave up breastfeeding within the first 4 months of delivery because they were returning to work (White et al 1992). This number has continued to rise, with 33% of those breastfeeding in 1995 giving up at 3–4 months because of employment commitments (Foster et al 1997) and 39% giving up between 4 and 6 months in 2000 (Hamlyn et al 2002). Several studies have found that a return to work is associated with early cessation of breastfeeding (Auerbach & Guss 1984, Barber-Madden et al 1987, Kearney & Cronenwett 1991, Ryan et al 2006, Simopoulos & Grave 1984, White et al 1992). An American study of middle-class mothers found that those in part-time employment breastfed their babies for longer than those in full-time employment (Fein & Roe 1998).

A recent American study (Ryan et al 2006) which collected data from a large national sample of new mothers (n = 228,000) investigated the initiation and duration of breastfeeding to 6 months among women who worked full time, part time or were not employed outside the home. Women who worked part time had a significantly higher uptake of breastfeeding than those who worked full time or were not employed, and working full time had a negative effect on breastfeeding duration. At 6 months after birth, 26.1% of women who worked full time were still breastfeeding, compared with 36.6% of women who worked part time and 35.0% who did not work. Stepwise multiple regression analysis of data for women who worked full time showed that combining full-time employment and breastfeeding was more likely to be achieved by women who had a normal birthweight infant, who were older, had a higher level of educational attainment and who were from Asian or white ethnic groups.

A return to employment after having a baby should not be seen as a barrier to the continuation of breastfeeding, but women may need guidance on how to combine breastfeeding with employment. No studies have investigated the content or effects of such guidance. A recent study from the UK (Kosmala-Anderson & Wallace 2006) determined the views and experiences of 46 employees in four large public sector organisations with regard to breastfeeding at work. The majority of women (80%) wanted to continue breastfeeding after returning to work; however, 90% were unaware of any employer policy nor were they offered information on support to enable breastfeeding after returning to work. This was despite two of the organisations having breastfeeding policies in development and some facilities in place. This is clearly an area which requires much more attention given the number of women returning to work and the short-term and longer term public health consequences of early cessation of breastfeeding.

## INFANT CONDITIONS THAT MAY AFFECT BREASTFEEDING

### Crying babies

A mother who is worried about her baby's crying may, as a result, doubt her ability to breastfeed and provide adequate nourishment for her baby. A mother may also be concerned that her baby has developed 'colic', a syndrome characterised by paroxysmal, excessive and inconsolable crying (Crowcroft & Strachan 1997), and may link this with breastfeeding. Little is known about risk factors for the development of colic generally, nor the effect of feeding method. As part of a large study of infant health during the first month of life in Sheffield, information on colic was collected from the parents of 67,172 infants born between 1975 and 1988 (Crowcroft & Strachan 1997); 12,277 (18.3%) infants were classed by parents as 'colicky' some time during the first month. Bottlefed infants were less likely to be reported as colicky, but after taking account of the stronger relationships of maternal age, parity and socio-economic circumstances, the excess among breastfed infants, although still statistically significant, was very much reduced (OR of breast compared with bottlefeeding 1.09, 95% CI 1.02–1.15).

Few studies have examined ways of preventing or treating crying or colic in breastfed babies. Woolridge & Fisher (1988), in a review of the feed management of babies with colic, proposed that babies may suffer colic as a result of incorrect feed management, and being taken off the breast before receiving sufficient quantities of hindmilk. As part of the trial by Evans et al (1995) referred to earlier, women were asked 6 months post delivery if their babies had colic (defined as episodes of inconsolable crying thought to be due to abdominal pain, and requiring medical advice). Of the 150 women in the group asked to carry out prolonged feeding from one breast, 19 (12%) reported colic, compared with 35 (23%) of the 152 women asked to feed from both breasts. Lucasson et al (1998) carried out a systematic review to evaluate the effectiveness of diets, drug treatments and behavioural interventions on infantile colic, with excessive crying or the presence of colic as the primary outcome measure; 27 trials fulfilled the inclusion criteria (interventions lasting at least 3 days in infants younger than 6 months who cried excessively). The results showed that elimination of cow's milk protein was effective when substituted by hypoallergenic formula milks, as was advice to reduce infant stimulation. The use of anticholinergic drugs showed some benefit but, due to reported side-effects, could not be recommended as treatment. A criticism of the review, however, is that the results of interventions in breast- and bottlefed babies were pooled, rather than being presented separately, so no conclusions relating specifically to breastfed infants can be drawn.

A Cochrane systematic review was undertaken to assess the effectiveness of infant massage in promoting infant physical and mental health (Underdown et al 2006). RCTs were included in which babies under the age of 6 months were randomised to an infant massage or a no-treatment control group, and which utilised a standardised outcome measure of infant mental or physical development. Twenty three studies were included in the review. The results of nine high-quality studies suggested that infant massage had no effect on growth, but provided some evidence suggestive of improved mother–infant interaction, sleep and relaxation, reduced crying and a beneficial impact on a number of hormones controlling stress. There was no evidence of effects on cognitive and behavioural outcomes, infant attachment or temperament. Data from 13 studies regarded as of lower quality showed uniformly significant benefits on growth, sleep, crying and bilirubin levels. The review authors concluded that the only evidence of a significant impact of massage on growth was obtained from this group of studies regarded to be at high risk of bias but there was some evidence of benefits on mother–infant interaction, sleeping and crying, and on hormones influencing stress levels. In the absence of evidence of harm, these findings may be sufficient to support the use of infant massage in the community, and may help women whose babies suffer from colic. Further research into massage as an effective intervention for babies with colic is required.

There remains insufficient research on ways to prevent or treat crying, for example to assess whether a change in feed management would reduce colic and stress in babies (Renfrew et al 2000). Research into the effect of the mother's diet (including smoking and a high caffeine intake) and non-pharmacological treatments, such as baby massage and support and education for parents, on a baby's crying is also required.

## Weight loss

The RCM handbook *Successful breastfeeding* states that 'in practice, the simplest and most readily applied "yardstick" is that the baby should have regained his birthweight by 10 days of age' (RCM 2002, p. 70). However, this will obviously rely on an accurate recording of the birthweight. It is questionable, however, whether growth standards that were based on infants who had largely been fed artificial milk should be applied to an exclusively breastfed baby (Whitehead & Paul 1985). A breastfed baby will initially grow more rapidly than a baby fed artificial milk during the first 2–3 months, a rate of gain which slows down at around 4 months.

## Jaundice

Physiological jaundice commonly presents in babies between 2 and 5 days old and as many as half of term babies develop this (Henschel & Inch 1996). Premature and/or low birthweight babies and those who are breastfed are more at risk. Breastfed babies tend to be at risk because human milk contains less vitamin K than artificial milk (Canfield et al 1991). Schneider (1986), in a review of 12 studies, found a higher incidence of jaundice in breastfed than bottlefed babies, but did not include details of when breastfeeding commenced or if babies were breastfed on demand. Most jaundice is benign but because of the potential toxicity of bilirubin, newborn infants must be monitored to identify those who might develop severe hyperbilirubinaemia. Jaundice before 24 hours of age is always considered pathological and requires immediate referral for further evaluation.

Vitamin K deficiency can cause bleeding in an infant in the first weeks of life, known as haemorrhagic disease of the newborn (HDN). HDN is divided into three categories: early, classic and late. Early HDN occurs within 24 hours of birth. Classic HDN occurs on days 1–7; common bleeding sites are gastrointestinal, cutaneous, nasal and from a circumcision. Late HDN occurs from weeks 2 to 12; the most common bleeding sites are intracranial, cutaneous and gastrointestinal. Late-onset HDN almost exclusively occurs in breastfed infants and in infants with liver disease or malabsorption. Vitamin K is commonly given prophylactically after birth for the prevention of HDN, although there have been concerns over route of administration which can be intramuscular (IM) or oral.

In 1992, Golding and colleagues reported an association between childhood cancer and IM administration of vitamin K. This finding was based upon a case–control study of 195 cases of childhood cancer and 558 controls. There was a significant association ($p = 0.002$) with childhood cancer and IM vitamin K (OR 1.97, CI 1.3–3.0) when compared with oral vitamin K or no vitamin K.

Following Golding's report, additional studies were conducted by other investigators which did not support a clinical relationship between newborn parenteral administration of vitamin K and childhood cancer. An expert group convened in October 1997 by the UK Medicines Control Agency on its own behalf and for the Department of Health and Committee of Safety of Medicines reviewed the studies linking vitamin K and childhood cancer. The Working Group considered eight case–control and four ecological studies and concluded that overall, the available data did not support an increased risk of cancer, including leukaemia, caused by vitamin K (Department of Health 1998).

A recently conducted large national UK Childhood Cancer Study (UKCCS) included an updated pooled analysis with data for 7017 children (1174 with leukaemia). It found no association between IM vitamin K and any diagnostic group, with a pooled odds ratio for leukaemia diagnosed between 12 and 71 months of age of 0.98 (CI 0.79–1.22) (Fear et al 2003). The authors concluded that in the light of all available evidence, chance was the most likely explanation for early findings regarding the link between vitamin K and childhood cancer.

A Cochrane systematic review was undertaken of prophylactic vitamin K for vitamin K deficiency bleeding in neonates (Puckett & Offringa 2000). Two eligible randomised trials, which compared a single dose of intramuscular vitamin K with placebo or nothing, assessed the effect on clinical bleeding. One dose of vitamin K reduced clinical bleeding at 1–7 days, including bleeding after circumcision, and improved biochemical indices of coagulation status. Eleven additional eligible randomised trials compared either a single oral dose of vitamin K with placebo or nothing, a single oral with a single IM dose of vitamin K, or three oral doses with a single intramuscular dose, but none assessed clinical bleeding. Oral vitamin K improved biochemical indices of coagulation status at 1–7 days. There was no evidence of a difference between the oral and IM route in effects on biochemical indices of coagulation status. A single oral compared with a single IM dose resulted in lower plasma vitamin K levels at 2 weeks and 1 month, whereas a three-dose oral schedule resulted in higher plasma vitamin K levels at 2 weeks and at 2 months than did a single IM dose.

The reviewers concluded that a single dose (1.0 mg) of IM vitamin K after birth is effective in the prevention of classic HDN. Either IM or oral (1.0 mg) vitamin K prophylaxis improves biochemical indices of coagulation status at 1–7 days. Neither IM nor oral vitamin K has been tested in randomised trials with respect to effect on late HDN.

The IM route was the most common route of administration of vitamin K until the publication by Golding et al (1992). Subsequently, the Royal College of Paediatrics and Child Health recommended that infants should receive vitamin K supplementation orally with several doses to be given to infants who were breastfed. Uncertainty about the optimum dosage led to variations in oral regimens in the UK. In addition, some inherent problems with oral dosing which potentially compromised effectiveness were identified.

These included compliance with a number of oral regimens and potential unreliability of absorption of oral vitamin K.

Current advice from the Department of Health continues to be that all newborn babies receive an appropriate vitamin K regimen to prevent the rare but serious and sometimes fatal disorder of HDN. Based on evidence of clinical and cost effectiveness, the NICE postnatal care guideline (NICE 2006) recommends that all babies receive a single dose of 1 mg IM. Parents who wish their infants to receive oral vitamin K should be aware of the importance of ensuring all doses are given.

## Ankyloglossia (tongue tie)

Tongue tie describes a condition arising when the sublingual frenulum (a fold of mucosa connecting the midline of the inferior surface of the tongue to the floor of the mouth) is unusually thick, tight or short (Hall & Renfrew 2005). Around 3–4% of infants may be affected (Hall & Renfrew 2005). The impact on the mobility of the tongue can have implications for women who wish to breastfeed their babies, including problems with latching, sore nipples, pain during feeding and, for the infant, failure to gain weight and unco-ordinated sucking (NICE 2005). Management options have included conservative approaches, such as advice on attachment on the breast, or surgical division of the frenulum.

Only one RCT has been conducted which compared outcomes of performing frenulectomy with conservative management (Hogan et al 2005), other data on outcomes coming from observational studies or case series (Fernando 1998, Messner et al 2000). Hogan et al (2005) identified 201 infants (11%) out of a cohort of 1866 live births with tongue tie, 57 (3%) of whom were randomised to division of the tongue tie (n = 28) or to a control group (n = 29). Main outcome measures included improvement in feeding as reported by the infant's mother. In the intervention group (which included both breast- and bottlefed infants), improvement in feeding within 48 hours was reported among 27 (96%) of the infants, compared with one (3%) of the infants in the control. When breastfeeding infants only were compared, 19 (95%) out of 20 infants were reported to have improved feeding in the intervention group, compared with one (5%) out of 20 in the control group, a significant difference (p<0.001). There were methodological problems with the trial, including lack of blinding of the mother and the investigator, and women of all babies in the control were offered division of tongue tie after 48 hours as it was considered unethical not to do so, thus limiting the opportunity to compare whether any babies improved spontaneously.

There continues to be limited evidence of the true prevalence of this condition, the most appropriate way to diagnose the condition and when this should be done. What is clear is that if women are having problems with breastfeeding, tongue tie should be considered as a potential cause.

Intervention procedure guidance produced by NICE on division of tongue tie (NICE 2005) has recommended that division be offered, given a lack of evidence of major safety concerns and potential to improve breastfeeding, and that the procedure should be performed by a healthcare professional who has been appropriately trained.

## SUMMARY OF THE EVIDENCE USED IN THIS GUIDELINE

- Evidence from a range of studies, including randomised controlled trials, has found that breast milk has many health advantages for the infant. Evidence of health advantages of breastfeeding for the woman is less conclusive.
- Evidence from a systematic review of interventions to promote the initiation of breastfeeding suggests that breastfeeding education will increase initiation among women on low incomes. As this evidence is based on US studies, the extent to which this would be found in other populations should be considered.
- Evidence from a systematic review suggests that skin-to-skin contact following birth may enhance breastfeeding uptake and duration with no evidence of harm, although studies were methodologically poor.
- There is evidence that structured programmes to support breastfeeding, such as the Baby Friendly Initiative, will increase the initiation of breastfeeding. The impact on duration is unclear and further research should be undertaken.
- Evidence from five RCTs and two non-RCTs has shown that supplements should not be given to breastfed babies unless medically indicated.
- Evidence from one large RCT, judged to be of good quality, has shown that flat or inverted nipples are not a contraindication to breastfeeding.
- Trial evidence is available to show that sore nipples should not be treated with topical preparations. Further evidence is required to determine the most effective management of this and other breastfeeding problems.
- A systematic review found high-quality evidence that additional postnatal support for exclusive and any breastfeeding is effective among women from relatively advantaged backgrounds. Evidence from studies of a lower quality which were targeted at women from disadvantaged backgrounds found that support can be effective for any feeding, but no evidence was found of effective interventions to support exclusive breastfeeding amongst this group.
- Evidence from a systematic review of the effectiveness of infant massage found no evidence of harm and potential benefits for mother–infant interaction, sleeping and crying and infant colic
- Evidence from a UK cohort study presenting data on over 7000 children does not support an increased risk of childhood cancer caused by IM administration of vitamin K.
- Evidence from one small but methodologically poor RCT supports division of infant tongue tie to improve breastfeeding.

## WHAT TO DO

### Support for breastfeeding

The NICE postnatal care guideline (NICE 2006) recommends the following.

- All maternity care providers should implement an externally evaluated, structured programme that encourages breastfeeding using the Baby Friendly Initiative as a minimum standard.
- Breastfeeding support should be made available regardless of the location of care.
- All women and their babies should have skin-to-skin contact as soon as possible following the birth.

### General advice for all breastfeeding women

- Within the first 24 hours of the birth, the physiology of lactation should be briefly outlined, including the mechanism of milk removal from the breast and the composition of breast milk. Sensitively explore the mother's knowledge of breastfeeding: the advice received, key issues such as when to feed, how to avoid problems and if necessary deal with them.
- The healthcare professional should ideally be present at a breastfeed to assist the mother to achieve good positioning (Fig. 4.1).

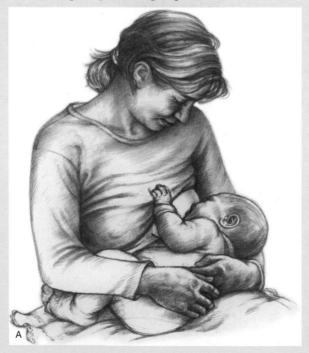

A

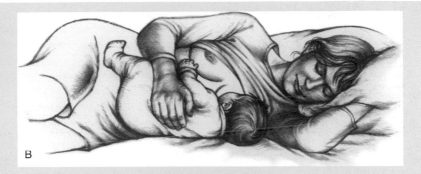

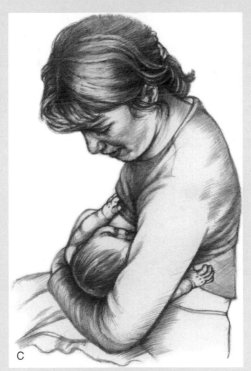

**Figure 4.1 A–C**   Nursing positions which could be adopted by the mother.

- Additional support with positioning and attachment should be offered to women who have had:
  - narcotic analgesia or general anaesthesia, as the baby may not initially be responsive to feeding
  - a caesarean section, particularly to assist with handling and positioning the baby to protect the woman's abdominal wound
  - initial contact with their baby delayed.

- When commencing a feed, the baby should be close to the mother, with his head and shoulders facing her breast and his nose at the same level as the nipple. The mother should allow the baby's top lip to touch the nipple until the baby gapes. The mother should then bring her baby quickly to the breast aiming his bottom lip as far as possible away from the nipple. The bottom lip will touch the breast first because the baby's head is extended (Fig. 4.2). This will ensure enough of the mother's breast is drawn into the baby's mouth to create a teat. When the baby commences suckling the mother may feel a strong 'drawing' sensation, but not sharp pain; the whole of the baby's lower jaw moves; she may hear the baby swallowing. A mother will be able to recognise if her baby is *nipple sucking* as she will feel pain; the baby will make frequent little sucks, will not change the rhythm of sucking and will not settle after a feed.
- If a feed is painful explain that this is probably due to the baby being incorrectly attached on the breast. The mother should gently take the baby off, then commence the feed again. Even if breast pain does not result in cessation of breastfeeding, discomfort can be considerable and last for many weeks. Appropriate and consistent midwifery advice can usually prevent or relieve this.
- A mother may initially need to support her breasts when positioning her baby to feed; once the baby is sucking, the support is usually no longer required
- Reassure that colostrum will totally meet the needs of the baby in the first few days after birth. Supplementary fluids are not needed unless medically indicated.
- Offer information about the nurturing benefits of putting the baby to the breast in addition to nutritional benefits.
- Advise women that they may experience difficulties attaching the baby at the breast when lactation starts (refer to section on 'engorgement'). Reassure them that they can contact a healthcare professional for help.
- Advise of the need for unrestricted feeding from one breast at a time when lactation commences, before feeding from the second breast, to ensure the baby receives both fore- and hindmilk.
- Explain that the baby will establish a sucking rhythm and does not need encouragement or stimulation to suck continuously. Feeding frequency may be variable over the first few days. When lactation is established, a baby will generally feed every 2–3 hours, but this will vary between babies. If the baby is healthy, his individual feeding pattern should be respected.

- As relatives can be negative about breastfeeding, involve the partner and other relatives who may help to care for the baby in discussions about the benefits of breastfeeding and ways to prevent and resolve problems. Where the views of relatives are negative, women may require additional midwifery support.
- Ensure that mothers have contact numbers for their healthcare professionals and local breastfeeding support groups to enable early assistance if a problem develops.

**Figure 4.2 A-C**   How to ensure the baby achieves correct positioning and attachment on the breast.

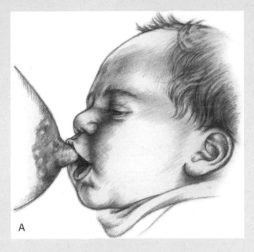

A

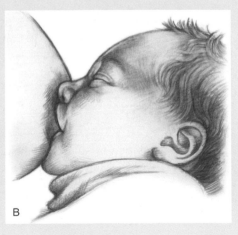

B

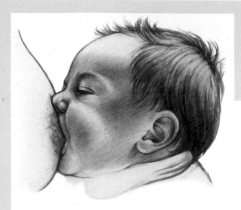

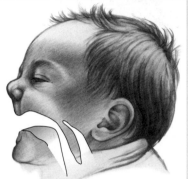

① nipple
② areola and breast tissue,
   with underlying milk ducts
③ baby's tongue
④ baby's throat

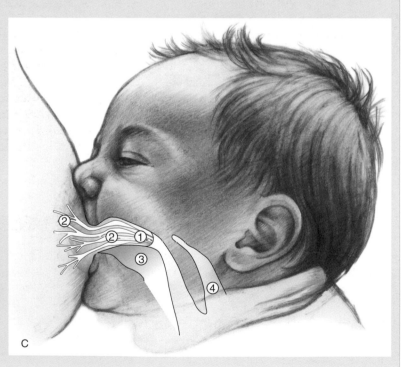

C

## Expressing breast milk

There are situations when mothers may need to express breast milk, e.g. if they have engorged breasts, for freezing breast milk supplies before recommencing employment, or to involve their partner in feeding. If mothers can express milk and go out occasionally without their baby, it could facilitate longer duration of breastfeeding. There has been concern that if a breastfed baby takes milk from a bottle, he will not 'remember' how to take the milk from the breast (sometimes referred to as 'nipple confusion') but there is no evidence to support this. All mothers should be taught how to express, once lactation has commenced. Some women may prefer to hand express, others to use electric pumps.

- **Preparation.** Some women may find initial attempts at expressing milk easiest in the bath or shower; warm flannels applied to the breasts may help to stimulate 'let-down'.
- **Timing of expressing.** The mother should express after a feed to generate 'extra' milk to store or to give to the baby later. If the baby usually only feeds from one breast, it may be helpful to express from the other breast at the same time, as lactation will be enhanced by the 'let-down' reflex. Reassure that expressing breast milk will not decrease the supply for the baby, but will increase the overall supply of milk
- **To hand express milk.** Gentle pressure should be exerted on the inner edge of the ampullae, by placing the forefinger at the lower edge of the areola and thumb at the upper edge. Using a steady rhythmic movement, the breast should be 'massaged', ensuring all lobes are emptied in rotation. The mother may be able to express milk directly into a sterilised bottle which can be stored for up to 24 hours in a fridge, but must be discarded after this. Expressed breast milk can be frozen for 1 week in a fridge freezer or up to 3 months in a deep freeze. Thawed milk should be discarded after 24 hours and breast milk never refrozen.

## Initial assessment

The purpose of this is to determine whether a mother is on course to breastfeed effectively or already has a problem. *Appropriate positioning and attachment on the breast and unrestricted feeding will prevent and resolve most breastfeeding problems.* Establish breastfeeding history. The following checklist is helpful when assessing how breastfeeding is progressing. Check with the mother that her baby:

- sucks deeply and rhythmically, with occasional pauses
- does not hurt her
- comes off the breast when he is ready
- during or after each feed, has the chance to wind.

The mother can be reassured, from the following checklist, that her breastfeeding is going well if her baby:

- grows steadily
- has straw coloured (pale yellow or clear), odourless urine
- has a regular, soft (but not totally liquid) yellow stool
- breastfeeds well and comes off on his own and looks satisfied.
  (Infant checklist taken from Renfrew et al (2004, p.106.)

Risk factors for potential breastfeeding problems (e.g. low birthweight and/or premature birth, multiple birth) should be considered when deciding upon the level of support a woman may require. Information for this initial assessment will also come from examination of the baby: jaundice +/-; hydrated +/-; drowsiness; weight gain.

At the end of this assessment the mother may be categorised in one of two ways.

### 1. On course to breastfeed effectively as planned

A mother says she is breastfeeding confidently, reports no breast problems, the baby finishes feeds spontaneously, is settling after feeds and physical examination of the baby suggests no problems. It is realistic, however, to advise that problems could still arise but these are manageable and should not necessitate stopping breastfeeding.

- Ask about breastfeeding goals: has she decided how long she will breastfeed or decided to 'see how it goes'?
- Arrange an appropriate revisit. For example, if a woman is first seen prior to lactation it would be appropriate to return by day 5 to check there are no problems.
- Provide information about local breastfeeding support groups.
- At each visit check on progress with breastfeeding and encourage continuation, ensuring consistent advice at all times.

### 2. Mother complains of breastfeeding problems

Obtain history: occurrence of problems in relation to feeding, mother's idea of cause. After discussion, examine the breasts, looking for nipple redness, cracks or bleeding; localised swelling of breasts, tenderness, redness. If she appears unwell take her temperature. If pyrexial, can this be related to a specific breast problem? Exclude other causes of infection and refer as appropriate (urgent action).

After history and examination it should be possible to classify problems into the following categories.

*Painful nipples*
A sharp, acute pain when the baby latches onto the breast is likely to be due to painful nipples and almost always is the result of incorrect attachment. The mother may also experience nipple or breast pain when she is not breastfeeding. There may be nipple redness, cracks or bleeding but should be no evidence of localised swelling, tenderness of the main breast or engorgement.

- Advice on the importance of effective positioning and attachment on the breast must be given.

- Advice on how to break suction gently with her forefinger when taking the baby off the breast may be helpful.
- There is no scientific evidence to support the use of creams, ointments or sprays or exposing the nipples to air, but they may provide temporary relief. It is probably better to advise the mother, if she wishes to apply some form of moisture, to rub expressed colostrum or breast milk on her nipples.
- Nipple shields are of limited value in resolving painful nipples, and should not be used before the mother has an established milk supply. If a mother is unable to feed because of severe nipple trauma, 'resting and expressing' over a 24-hour period may reduce the trauma (refer to Expressing breast milk, p. 90, for guidance on this).
- After 24 hours, the healthcare professional should help the mother to recommence direct breastfeeding, ensuring that this is pain free. If the nipples are still painful, positioning and attachment should be checked again.
- The mother should be reassured that once positioning and attachment are effective, the nipples will heal very quickly. If the nipple pain persists after repositioning and reattachment have been assessed, assessment for thrush should be considered.

### Engorgement

This symptom is common when lactation commences, usually 2–3 days after delivery. Both breasts can be affected. Signs are red, tender and full breasts. There should be no signs of localised swelling. There may be a mild pyrexia, tachycardia and flu-like symptoms. Engorgement which occurs after this may result from the mother missing feeds, but the same advice should be given.

- Unrestricted feeding and effective positioning and attachment will prevent and/or relieve this.
- If the areola is engorged, the mother may need to be shown how to express sufficient milk to soften the areola to enable the baby to latch on (refer to Expressing breast milk, p. 90).
- Analgesia may be required (paracetamol should be recommended).
- Ensure that an obstruction in the breast is not caused by a badly fitting bra.
- Be aware that if engorgement is not relieved the woman may develop mastitis.

### Insufficient milk

A mother may express concern that because her baby is not settling after a feed, is waking frequently for feeds or is not gaining weight, she is not providing adequate milk. This is one of the most commonly reported reasons for giving up breastfeeding.

- Reassure that this can almost always be dealt with since actual (rather than perceived) insufficient milk is extremely rare.
- Mothers should be aware of the importance of effective positioning and attachment on the breast to aid the establishment of lactation.

- Mothers should not limit the duration of feeds: the baby should empty the first breast before going to the second. After the milk is 'in' it is important that the baby is able to empty the breast of fore- and hindmilk at each feed.
- It may be helpful to suggest different feeding positions (refer to p. 86).
- If appropriate feeding practices do not alleviate the problem and there are concerns about the mother's milk supply and/or the baby's growth, referral should be made (urgent action).
- Encourage and support the mother to continue breastfeeding. Do not recommend that the baby receives supplementary fluids until all efforts to establish breastfeeding have been made. If supplementary fluids do become necessary, expressed breast milk should be given by a cup or a bottle.

*Thrush*

The mother may complain of a burning sensation or deep breast pain, lasting for several minutes during or after a feed. The skin on the nipples and areola may be red, itchy and shiny. There should be no evidence of localised swelling. The baby should be examined for signs of oral or perianal thrush. Referral should be made for a prescription (urgent action).

- Contacts should be planned to check symptoms are responding.
- The mother may require pain relief when feeding, until antifungal treatments take effect.
- If symptoms do not respond in either mother or baby, or if recurrence is suspected, refer back (urgent action).
- The mother should be advised about the need to wash her hands following each nappy change, to change breast pads frequently and to wear cotton underwear.

*Blocked milk duct*

The mother will be generally well, but will complain of a localised lump or tenderness, usually in one breast. This can occur at any time throughout the breastfeeding period.

- Advise on the importance of a well-fitting bra. Varying feeding positions may help to relieve the blocked duct (refer to Initial Assessment section).
- Explain how to 'milk' the breast to relieve pressure on the blocked duct (refer to the RCM's 2002 publication *Successful breastfeeding*, p.105).
- Advise about the possibility of developing mastitis and the importance of adhering to primary intervention measures to avoid this.
- Visits to assess progress should be made. If a mother has a breast lump which does not resolve after appropriate management, she should be referred for further assessment.

*Inverted or non-protractile nipples*

A mother with inverted or non-protractile nipples may experience difficulty achieving effective positioning of her baby on the breast, and should receive extra support and care to ensure successful breastfeeding.

- Reassure the mother that she is likely to achieve successful breastfeeding, as babies *breast* feed and do not *nipple* feed, but she will need more patience and help.
- The baby should be encouraged to take a large mouthful of breast tissue. The baby will help to draw the nipple out by sucking.
- It may help women to stimulate their nipples with their fingers, prior to a feed, to help them stand out.
- If, during the first few days of delivery, problems are experienced with direct breastfeeding, lactation may be initiated using a breast pump and the milk fed to the baby with a cup or a spoon. Once the milk is 'in' and the breasts have softened, further attempts at direct breastfeeding should be made. After a couple of weeks of expressing breast milk, the baby is likely to be able to breastfeed successfully as the nipples may have been drawn out.
- If only one breast is affected, the mother could feed the baby from the unaffected breast and express milk from the other.

*Mastitis (non-infective)*
Mastitis commonly presents as a red, tender lump, usually in one breast. The mother may complain of flu-like symptoms and may have a history of blocked milk duct. She may or may not have a pyrexia.

- Ensure that the breast is emptied at each feed. If the mother has been unable to feed because of painful nipples, refer to relevant section for management.
- The baby will need to feed from the affected breast first as the sucking of a hungry baby should encourage drainage. Frequent feeds will keep the breasts from becoming overly full.
- Advise the mother that she can take analgesia (paracetamol) prior to the feed to alleviate discomfort.
- As with a blocked duct, the mother should gently massage the lump whilst the baby is feeding to help relieve the pressure.
- Visit frequency should be discussed with the mother, but regular visits should be made to ensure that the mother is confident about her management of the symptom.
- Encourage bed rest and plenty of fluids until the flu-like symptoms have resolved.
- The mother should not stop breastfeeding, as this could exacerbate the symptom.
- If these measures do not ease symptoms within a few hours, referral must be made to prevent the possibility of mastitis infection and abscess; antibiotic therapy may be needed (urgent action).
- Increased frequency of midwifery visits should be planned to give breastfeeding support and to observe mother and baby for signs of thrush if antibiotics are taken.

*Mastitis (infective)/breast abscess*
The mother will report a history of sudden onset, flu-like symptoms and pyrexia. Cellulitis in a breast lobe or erythema around the areola may also be noted. The breast will be swollen, red and hot with intense localised pain. This may occur

following ineffective or delayed treatment for mastitis or staphylococcal infection from a cracked nipple. If symptoms of mastitis are not treated, a breast abscess may develop.

- **Urgent action is necessary.**
- A mother with infective mastitis will require antibiotics and analgesia, bed rest and plenty of fluids until flu-like symptoms have resolved.
- She should be advised to continue breastfeeding (providing there is no pus), or express the milk. The milk must not be left in the breast as, even with the use of antibiotics, an abscess could develop.
- If a breast abscess is suspected, it is likely that the mother will require referral to hospital when aspiration of the abscess will be undertaken as first-line treatment, followed by a course of antibiotics.
- If pus is draining from the nipple, feeding could continue from the unaffected breast.
- Contacts should be planned to ensure the prescribed treatment regimen is effective and to offer support.

### Women who may require additional breastfeeding support

#### Multiple births

At the initial home visit, reassurance should be given that the supply and demand physiology of lactation will enable the mother to provide sufficient milk for her infants.

- Practice suggests that the mother will benefit from adopting a regular feeding routine (not recommended for single infants), and if possible feed the infants at the same time, as this will enable her to rest. Feeding at the same time will also maintain prolactin levels.
- The mother may require additional advice on feeding positions.
- Contact numbers for local multiple birth support groups should be given.

#### Mothers who wish to combine breastfeeding with a return to work

Advice should be appropriate to the timing of the return to employment. Information on how to express and store breast milk is essential (refer to Expressing breast milk, p. 90). The National Childbirth Trust and La Leche League provide advice on combining work and continuing breastfeeding but women need to know how to contact these groups.

- If a mother expresses milk during the early weeks of breastfeeding this can be frozen and stored in sterile containers with airtight tops.
- All stored milk should be labelled with date and time of collection. It can be stored in a fridge for up to 24 hours, or kept in a deep freezer for up to 3 months.

- Although not evidence based, current practice is that any thawed milk should be discarded within 24 hours if unused or if it has been in contact with the baby's saliva.
- Mothers can express milk several times a day. Different methods of expressing milk can be attempted to find the most suitable.

## Infant conditions that may affect breastfeeding

### Crying

The mother is likely to be anxious and find it difficult to cope with a baby who cries a lot. She may be concerned that her baby is hungry or has colic. However, it is difficult to distinguish this from other signs of distress in the baby.

- Observe the mother feeding to check that she has adopted an effective breastfeeding technique.
- Check that the baby feeds for long enough on the breast to take sufficient hindmilk.
- Reassure that she will learn the difference between crying for a feed and crying for another reason. Babies cry for other reasons, not just when they are hungry. A new baby will usually have a good feed if he is hungry.
- Ask the mother about the colour of the baby's stools.
- Ask the mother *when* the baby cries and the duration of crying; if it happens after a good feed, the baby may have wind. Advise on how to wind the baby. She should check if the nappy needs changing.
- Baby massage may soothe the baby and advice on how to seek guidance on undertaking massage should be given. Calming music and walking in rhythm may also help. If the baby does not stop, advise the mother to let him cry but cuddle him. Try to get the woman's partner or another relative to help.
- Ask if the mother has altered her diet as some foods may cause a reaction in the baby. If she smokes or has a high caffeine intake, advise her to cut down or stop as these could be causing a sensitivity in the baby.
- Before a feed, the mother should try to calm herself, perhaps by asking her partner or relative/friend to take the baby for a few minutes. Reassure that a baby who continues to cry for no apparent reason is just as likely to cry if bottlefed.
- If a baby continues to have episodes of inconsolable crying but is otherwise healthy, it may be helpful to refer the mother to a voluntary support group such as CRY-SIS.
- If there are any concerns about the well-being of the baby or the mother, referral should be made (urgent action).

### Weight loss

As a general rule the baby should have regained his birthweight by 10 days of age. Weight gain should be used as one of the indicators that the baby is healthy (refer to Infant Checklist, Initial Assessment section).

- The baby should be weighed on the same scales throughout the postnatal period. Accurate information should be given to the mother, to avoid confusion. In the absence of trial evidence on weighing frequency, if there are concerns about the baby's weight and overall condition, weigh daily.
- The baby should be weighed naked, before a feed and at the same time of day, to minimise fluctuations.
- If weight gain is static or there is concern about weight loss, ensure the baby is effectively positioned on the breast and feeding duration is not limited. If a mother has no breastfeeding problems, she can be advised that she can supplement the occasional feed with a bottle, but only if lactation is established.
- If there is any concern about the baby's condition, taking other indicators of health into account, referral should be made (urgent action).

### Jaundice

Physiological jaundice may occur within 2–5 days of delivery. The baby's skin will have a yellow hue, he may be sleepy and the mother is likely to report that he is not feeding well. Stools may be green.

- Ensure the baby receives vitamin K prophylaxis according to local protocol. NICE recommends that all babies should receive a single dose of 1 mg IM vitamin K; if parents wish their baby to have oral prophylaxis, they should be aware of the need to ensure that all doses are administered in accordance with the manufacturer's instructions.
- Reassure the mother that this symptom is common among breastfeeding babies.
- The baby should receive regular (at least 3 hourly) feeds.
- If jaundice develops in babies aged 24 hours or older, its intensity should be monitored and systematically recorded along with the baby's overall well-being, with particular regard to hydration and alertness.
- Arrange a visit to coincide with a feed to assist the mother in putting the baby to the breast. Ensure that the baby is well positioned to receive colostrum, which acts as a laxative and will help the baby to pass meconium.
- If the milk is 'in', emphasise the importance of the baby receiving hindmilk, as the higher fat content is more effective at stimulating bowel evacuation.
- Fluid supplements should not be given.
- Blood should be taken for a serum bilirubin and appropriate referral made if symptoms are progressive and do not respond to effective breastfeeding practice (urgent action).
- Every effort should be made to prevent separation of mother and baby if phototherapy is required.
- If jaundice first develops after 7 days or remains after 14 days in an otherwise healthy baby and a cause has not already been identified, it should be evaluated (urgent action).

### Tongue tie

Women may report problems with breastfeeding, in attaching their baby to the breast, unco-ordinated sucking, sore nipples, breast pain during a feed or concerns about their baby failing to put on weight.

- All potential causes should be investigated in the first instance, including observation for correct attachment on the breast and unrestricted feeding.
- If tongue tie is suspected, referral should be made for further assessment and management (urgent action).

## SUMMARY GUIDELINE

## Breastfeeding issues

### Initial assessment – All breastfeeding women

- Evaluate breastfeeding:
  - on course to feed effectively
  - problem already present
- Ask about the behaviour of the baby
- Assess knowledge and give general advice as appropriate

### Urgent action is required if:

- Maternal or infant thrush
- Infective mastitis
- Breast abscess
- Concern about baby's well-being
- Concern about onset and/or severity of jaundice

## What to do

### Painful nipples

- Assess positioning and attachment of baby on the breast
- Advise mother of appropriate nursing position
- No evidence to justify use of creams, ointments or sprays
- Further visit(s) to review

## Engorgement

- If areola engorged, mother may need to express milk before a feed
- Pain relief (paracetamol) may be required
- Unrestricted feeding will help relieve problem
- If engorgement is not relieved the mother may develop mastitis
- Further visit(s) to review

## Insufficient milk

- Reassure that this can almost always be dealt with
- Discuss importance of positioning and attachment of baby on breast
- Emphasise importance of baby taking fore- and hindmilk
- There should be no limit on the duration of feeds
- If above do not solve the problem and there is concern about baby's growth, refer (urgent action)

## Thrush/infective mastitis/breast abscess

- After referral, outcomes of treatment should be reviewed

## Blocked milk duct

- Show mother how to 'milk' the duct
- Discuss different feeding positions
- Advise re possibility of developing mastitis
- Further visit(s) to review

## Non-infective mastitis

- Advise analgesia (paracetamol) prior to feed
- Feed from affected side first
- Frequent feeds
- Encourage bed rest, until flu-like symptoms have resolved
- If symptoms not eased in 6–8 hours (telephone to find out), refer (urgent action)
- If symptoms have eased, increase visit frequency until resolved

**Inverted or non-protractile nipples**

- Reassure mother that babies breastfeed and do not 'nipple' feed
- If only one breast is affected, feed from the unaffected side
- If initial problems experienced with direct breastfeeding, initiate lactation with breast pump and feed baby with cup or spoon. Direct breastfeed when milk is 'in'

**General advice**

- Avoid conflicting advice
- Emphasise the importance of correct positioning and attachment of the baby on the breast
- Advise about different nursing positions; as long as correct positioning and attachment on the breast are achieved, no one position is better than another
- If suckling causes pain take the baby off the breast, reposition and reattach
- Reassure that colostrum will fully meet the needs of the baby, and supplementary feeds are not necessary
- Emphasise the importance of unrestricted feeding on demand
- Include partner and any close relatives involved in care of the baby in discussion of breastfeeding advantages
- If problem develops, midwife can be contacted
- Provide addresses/telephone numbers of local breastfeeding support groups

## Advice on hand expressing breast milk

- Advise the woman to practise hand expressing before stored supplies are required, for example, before she recommences employment. As the mother becomes more confident, she may find other ways of expressing milk which she feels are better for her
- To hand express, the mother should place her thumb flat on the upper edge of the areola and cup the rest of her hand under her breast. Her forefinger should rest on the lower edge of the areola. She should then gently squeeze her thumb and forefinger together, and at the same time, gently press her whole hand back and in, towards the chest wall. Doing these movements together enables milk from the deep breast tissue to be expressed as well as the ducts beneath the areola and nipple

## References

Alexander J, Grant A, Campbell M 1992 RCT of breast shells and Hoffman's exercises for inverted and non-protractile nipples. BMJ 304: 1030-1032

Amir L 1991 Candida and the lactating breast: predisposing factors. J Hum Lactation 7: 171-181

Amir L, Forster D, McLachlan H et al 2004 Incidence of breast abscess in lactating women: report from an Australian cohort. Br J Obstet Gynaecol 111: 1378-1381

Anderson G, Moore E, Hepworth J et al 2003 Early skin-to-skin contact for mothers and their healthy newborn infants. Cochrane Database of Systematic Reviews, Issue 3

Arenz S, Ruckerl R, Koletzko B et al 2004 Breastfeeding and childhood obesity: a systematic review. Int J Obesity 28: 1247-1256

Auerbach K, Guss E 1984 Maternal employment and breastfeeding. Am J Dis Child 138: 958-960

Barber-Madden R, Petschek M, Pakter J 1987 Breast feeding and the working mother: barriers and intervention strategies. J Public Health Policy 8: 531-541

Bartington S, Griffiths L, Tate A et al 2006 Are breastfeeding rates higher among mothers delivering in Baby Friendly accredited maternity units in the UK? Int J Epidemiology 35(5): 1178-1186

Bick DE, MacArthur C, Lancashire R 1998 What influences the uptake and early cessation of breast feeding? Midwifery 14: 242-247

Bolling K, Grant C, Hamlyn B et al 2007 Infant feeding survey 2005. BMRB Social Research, London

Broadfoot M, Britten J, Tappin DM et al 2005 The Baby Friendly Hospital Initiative and breast feeding rates in Scotland. Arch Dis Child Fetal Neonatal Ed 90(2): F114-116

Brown S, Lumley J 1997 Reasons to stay, reasons to go: results of an Australian population-based survey. Birth 24(3): 148-158

Brown S, Small R, Faber B et al 2002 Early postnatal discharge from hospital for healthy mothers and term infants. Cochrane Database of Systematic Reviews, Issue 3

Burr M, Miskelly F, Butland B et al 1989 Environmental factors and symptoms in infants at high risk of allergy. J Epidemiol Commun Health 43: 125-132

Canfield L, Hopkinson J, Lima A et al 1991 Vitamin K in colostrum and mature human milk over the lactation period – a cross sectional study. Am J Clin Nutr 53: 730-735

Carfoot S, Williamson P, Dickson R 2005 A randomised controlled trial in the north of England examining the effects of skin-to-skin care on breast feeding. Midwifery 21: 71-79

Cattaneo A, Buzzette R 2001 Effect on rates of breast feeding of training for the baby friendly hospital initiative – quality improvement report. BMJ 323(7325): 1358-1362

Cloherty M, Alexander J, Holloway I 2004 Supplementing breast-fed babies in the UK to protect their mothers from tiredness or distress. Midwifery 20(2): 194-204

Crowcroft N, Strachan D 1997 The social origins of infantile colic: questionnaire study covering 76,747 infants. BMJ 314: 1325-1328

Department of Health 1994 Weaning and the weaning diet. HMSO, London

Department of Health 1995 Breastfeeding: good practice guidance to the NHS. HMSO, London

Department of Health 1998 Department of Health, Nutrition and Bone Health COMA Expert Group. Report on Health and Social Subjects 49. HMSO, London

Department of Health 2003 Priorities and planning framework 2003–2006. Stationery Office, London

Department of Health 2004 National Service Framework for Children, Young People and the Maternity Services. Stationery Office, London

Deveraux W 1969 Acute puerperal mastitis. Evaluation of its management. Am J Obstet Gynecol 108(1): 78-81

DiGirolamo A, Grummer-Strawn L, Fein S 2001 Maternity care practices: implications for breastfeeding. Birth 28(2): 94-100

Dixon J 1988 Repeated aspiration of breast abscesses in lactating women. BMJ 297: 1517-1518

Duffy E, Percival P, Kershaw E 1997 Positive effects of an antenatal group teaching session on postnatal nipple pain, nipple trauma and breast feeding rates. Midwifery 13(4): 189-196

Dyson L, McCormick F, Renfrew MJ 2005 Interventions for promoting the initiation of breastfeeding. Cochrane Database of Systematic Reviews, Issue 2

Dyson L, Renfrew M, McFadden A et al 2006 Promotion of breastfeeding initiation and duration. Evidence into practice briefing. National Institute for Health and Clinical Excellence, London

Enkin M, Keirse M, Renfrew M et al 2000 A guide to effective care in pregnancy and childbirth, 3rd edn. Oxford University Press, Oxford

Eryilmaz R, Sahin M, Hakan Tekelioglu M et al 2005 Management of lactational breast abscesses. Breast 14(5): 375-379

Evans K, Evans R, Simmer K 1995 Effect of the method of breast feeding on breast engorgement, mastitis and infantile colic. Acta Paediatr 84(8): 849-852

Fear N, Roman E, Ansell P et al 2003 Vitamin K and childhood cancer: a report from the United Kingdom Childhood Cancer Study. Br J Cancer 89(7): 1228-1231

Fein S, Roe B 1998 The effect of work status on initiation and duration of breastfeeding. Am J Public Health 88: 1042-1046

Fernando C 1998 Tongue-tie – from confusion to clarity. Tandem, Sydney, Australia

Fewtrell M 2004 The long-term benefits of having been breast-fed. Curr Paediatr 14: 97-103

Foster K, Lader D, Cheesbrough S 1997 Infant feeding 1995, HMSO, London

Foxman B, D'Arcy H, Gillespie B et al 2002 Lactation mastitis: occurrence and medical management among 946 breastfeeding women in the United States. Am J Epidemiol 155: 103-114

Golding J, Greenwood R, Birmingham K et al 1992 Childhood cancer, intramuscular vitamin K and pethidine given in labour. BMJ 305: 341-346

Hall D, Renfrew M 2005 Tongue tie. Arch Dis Child 90: 1211-1215

Hally M, Bond J, Crawley J et al 1984 Factors influencing the feeding of first born infants. Acta Paediatr 73: 33-39

Hamelin K, McLennan J 2000 Examination of the use of an in-hospital breastfeeding assessment tool. Mother Baby J 5(3): 29-37

Hamlyn B, Brooker S, Oleinikova K et al 2002 Infant feeding 2000. Stationery Office, London

Henley S, Anderson C, Avery M et al 1995 Anemia and insufficient milk in first-time mothers. Birth 22(2): 87-92

Henschel D, Inch S 1996 Breastfeeding: a guide for midwives. Books for Midwives Press, Hale, Cheshire

Hoddinott P, Pill R 1999 Qualitative study of decisions about infant feeding among women in east end of London. BMJ 318: 30-34

Hogan M, Westcott C, Griffiths M 2005 A randomised controlled trial of tongue-tie in infants with feeding problems. J Paediatr Child Health 41: 242

Howie P, Forsyth J, Ogston S et al 1990 Protective effect of breast feeding against infection. BMJ 300: 11-16

Inch S, Fisher C 1999 Breast feeding. In: Marsh G, Renfrew M (eds) Community-based maternity care. Oxford University Press, Oxford

Kearney M, Cronenwett L 1991 Breast feeding and employment. J Gynaecol Neonatal Nurs 20: 471-480

Kinlay J, O'Connell D, Kinlay S 1998 Incidence of mastitis in breastfeeding women six months after delivery: a prospective cohort study. Med J Aust 169(6): 310-312

Kosmala-Anderson J, Wallace L 2006 Breastfeeding works: the role of employers in supporting women who wish to breastfeed and work in four organisations in England. J Public Health 28(3): 183-191

Kramer MS, Chalmers B, Hodnett E et al 2001 Promotion of Breastfeeding Intervention Trial (PROBIT): a randomised trial in the Republic of Belarus. JAMA 285(4): 413-420

Lathouwer de S, Lionet C, Lansac J et al 2004 Predictive factors of early cessation of breastfeeding. A prospective study in a university hospital. Eur J Obstet 117: 169-173

Lawrence R 1994 Breastfeeding – a guide for the medical profession, 4th edn. Mosby, New York

Loh N, Kelleher C, Long S et al 1997 Can we increase breast feeding rates? Irish Med J 90 (3): 100-101

Lucassen P, Assendelft W, Gubbels J et al 1998 Effectiveness of treatments for infantile colic: systematic review. BMJ 316:1563-1569

MAIN Trial Collaborative Group 1994 Preparing for breast feeding: treatment of inverted and non-protractile nipples in pregnancy. Midwifery 10(4): 200-214

Marild S, Jodal U, Hanson L 1990 Breastfeeding and urinary tract infection. Lancet 336: 942

Marild S, Hansson S, Jodal U et al 2004 Protective effect of breastfeeding against urinary tract infection. Acta Paediatr Scand 93(2): 164-168

McGeorge D 1994 The 'Niplette': an instrument for the non-surgical correction of inverted nipples. Br J Plast Surg 47(1): 46-49

Messner A, Lalakea M, Aby J et al 2000 Ankyloglossia: incidence and associated feeding difficulties. Arch Otolaryngeal Head Neck Surg 126: 36-39

Morrow A, Guerrero M, Shults J et al 1999 Efficacy of home-based peer counselling to promote exclusive breastfeeding: a randomised controlled trial. Lancet 353(9160): 1226-1231

National Institute for Health and Clinical Excellence 2005 Interventional Procedure Guidance (IPG)149. Division of ankyloglossia (tongue tie) for breastfeeding

National Institute for Health and Clinical Excellence 2006 Postnatal Care: Routine postnatal care of women and their babies. NICE Clinical Guideline 37

Neifert M, Seacat J, Jobe W 1986 Lactation failure due to insufficient glandular development of the breast. Paediatrics 76: 823-828

Oddy W, Holt P, Sly P et al 1999 Association between breast feeding and asthma in 6 year old children: findings of a prospective birth cohort study. BMJ 319: 815-819

O'Hara R, Dexter S, Fox J 1996 Conservative management of infective mastitis and breast abscesses after ultrasonographic assessment. Br J Surg 83(10): 1413-1414

Philipp B, Merewood A, Miller L et al 2001 Baby-friendly hospital initiative improves breastfeeding initiation rates in a US hospital setting. Pediatrics 108(3): 677-681

Pollard D 1998 Effect of self-regulation on breastfeeding in primiparous mothers. Thesis, University of Pittsburgh

Puckett RM, Offringa M 2000 Prophylactic vitamin K for vitamin K deficiency bleeding in neonates. Cochrane Database of Systematic Reviews, Issue 4

Radzyminski S 2003 The effect of ultra low dose epidural analgesia on newborn feeding behaviours. J Obstet Gynecol Neonatal Nurs 32: 322-331

Rajan L 1994 The impact of obstetric procedures and analgesia/anaesthesia during labour and delivery on breast feeding. Midwifery 10: 87-103

Ransjö-Arvidson A, Matthiesen A, Lilja G et al 2001 Maternal analgesia during labour disturbs newborn behaviour: effects on breastfeeding, temperature and crying. Birth 28(1): 5-12

Renfrew M, Woolridge M, Ross McGill H 2000 Enabling women to breast feed. A structured review of the evidence. Stationery Office, London

Renfrew M, Fisher C, Arms S 2004 Bestfeeding: getting breastfeeding right for you. Celestial Arts, Berkeley, California

Renfrew M, Dyson L, Wallace L et al 2005 The effectiveness of public health interventions to promote the duration of breastfeeding. National Institute for Health and Clinical Excellence, London

Royal College of Midwives (RCM) 2002 Successful breastfeeding, 3rd edn. Churchill Livingstone, Edinburgh

Ryan A S, Wenjun Z, Arensberg B 2006 The effect of employment status on breastfeeding in the United States. Women's Health Issues 16(5): 243-251

Sadauskaite-Kuehne V, Ludvigsson J, Pagaiga Z et al 2004 Longer breastfeeding is an independent protective factor against development of type 1 diabetes mellitus in childhood. Diabetes Metab Res Rev 20(2): 150-157

Schneider A 1986 Breast milk and jaundice in the newborn – a real entity. JAMA 225: 3270-3274

Simopoulos A, Grave G 1984 Factors associated with the choice and duration of infant feeding practice. Pediatrics 74(4): 603-614

Torvaldsen S, Roberts C, Simpson J et al 2006 Intrapartum epidural analgesia and breastfeeding: a prospective cohort study. Int Breastfeeding J 1: 24

Underdown A, Barlow J, Chung V et al 2006 Massage intervention for promoting mental and physical health in infants aged under six months. Cochrane Database of Systematic Reviews, Issue 4

Volmanen P, Valanne J, Alahuhta S 2004 Breast-feeding problems after epidural analgesia for labour: a retrospective cohort study of pain, obstetrical procedures and breast-feeding practices. Int J Obstet Anesth 13: 25-29

Waldenström U, Aarts C 2004 Duration of breastfeeding and breastfeeding problems in relation to length of postpartum stay: a longitudinal cohort study of a national Swedish sample. Acta Paediatr 93(5): 669-676

White A, Freeth S, O'Brien M 1992 Infant feeding 1990. A survey carried out for the DHSS by the Office of Population Censuses and Surveys. HMSO, London

Whitehead R, Paul A 1985 Growth charts and the assessment of infant feeding practices in the western world and in developing countries. Early Hum Dev 9: 187-207

Widstrom A, Wahlberg V, Matthiesen A et al 1990 Short-term effects of early sucking and touch of the nipple on maternal behaviour. Early Hum Dev 21: 153-163

Woolridge M, Fisher C 1988 Colic "overfeeding" and symptoms of lactose malabsorption in the breastfed baby: a possible artifact of feed management? Lancet 2: 382-384

World Health Organization (WHO) 2002 Infant and young child nutrition; global strategy for infant and young child feeding. World Health Organization, Geneva

Chapter **5**

# Urinary problems

---

**CHAPTER CONTENTS**

---

## INTRODUCTION

Stress incontinence is the most common of the urinary problems that occur in childbearing women, both in pregnancy and postpartum. Since the first edition of this book research on postpartum urinary stress incontinence has increased substantially. Urge incontinence, urinary retention/voiding difficulties and fistulae can also occur, although the latter are rare in developed countries and will not be reviewed in this guideline.

## URINARY INCONTINENCE

### Definition

Urinary incontinence includes stress incontinence, urge incontinence and mixed incontinence. The term 'stress incontinence' can be used either to describe a symptom or as a medical diagnosis. When describing a symptom it refers to the involuntary leakage of urine, usually on exertion or on sneezing or coughing (Abrams et al 2002). As a diagnosis it refers to involuntary loss of urine when the intravesical pressure exceeds that of the urethra, with no simultaneous detrusor contraction. The International Continence Society refer to the latter as 'genuine stress incontinence', but this diagnosis should only be made following urodynamic investigation (Cardozo & Khullar 1995). The definition of stress incontinence used in this chapter, unless otherwise specified, refers to a symptom rather than a diagnosis. Urge incontinence is the complaint of involuntary leakage accompanied by or immediately preceded by urgency (Abrams et al 2002). Some women have mixed incontinence, which is a combination of the two. Most studies of incontinence in postpartum women are of stress incontinence, which is the most common childbirth-related type, but some do not specify type and a few separately distinguish stress and urge incontinence.

## Frequency of occurrence

The prevalence of incontinence in the general female population varies according to the definition used and the age groups included, but it is very common (Yarnell et al 1981, Burgio et al 1991, O'Brien et al 1991, Hannestad et al 2000). Many observational studies have now examined the prevalence of urinary incontinence in postpartum women, again with variations in prevalence according to timing and methods of ascertainment. Some studies have assessed women over time and have found many symptoms to be persistent.

In a cross-sectional study of 1505 women in New Zealand, contacted by postal questionnaire at 3 months postpartum, 23.9% reported stress incontinence and a further 10.4% reported urge incontinence (Wilson et al 1996). A UK postal questionnaire survey of 11,701 women contacted 1–9 years after birth found that 20.6% reported stress incontinence that had started for the first time within 3 months of the delivery and lasted beyond 6 weeks (MacArthur et al 1991). Three-quarters of the symptomatic women reported symptoms lasting for at least 1 year.

A large multicentre longitudinal study recruited 7879 women at 3 months postpartum and 4214 were followed up at 6 years (MacArthur et al 2006). Of the women contacted at 6 years, 24% had urinary incontinence at both times (most had stress or mixed incontinence); of those who had been symptomatic when first contacted at 3 months, 73% still had symptoms.

Prevalence of urinary incontinence at 6 months postpartum in a Canadian cross-sectional study of 2492 primiparous women, with ascertainment using a postal questionnaire continence severity score index, was 29.6% (Hatem et al 2005). Type of incontinence was also ascertained, showing that 43% of symptomatic women had stress incontinence, 6% had urge, 13% had mixed, and for the remaining 38% type was unspecified. Farrell et al (2001), also in a Canadian study, recruited 690 primiparae and contacted them up to 6 months postpartum, when prevalence of urinary incontinence (type not specified) was 26%.

A national cohort study in Sweden (Schytt et al 2004), of 2390 women followed from early pregnancy using postal questionnaires, found prevalence of stress incontinence to be 22% at 12 months postpartum. Burgio et al (2003) in a US cohort study, following a convenience sample of 523 women just after birth and at 6 weeks, 3, 6 and 12 months, found prevalence of urinary incontinence (type not specified) ascertained by telephone interview at 12 months after birth to be 13.3%. Prevalence at the various contact points was very similar.

In an Australian study of 1336 women sent postal questionnaires at 6–7 months postpartum, prevalence of stress incontinence was 11% (Brown & Lumley 1998). This was lower than in most other studies but the wording of the questionnaire was whether their stress incontinence had been 'a problem' for them, and there is evidence to suggest that postpartum women do not always consider stress incontinence to be a problem (see below). Another Australian study contacted 1295 women immediately postpartum and at 8, 16 and 24 weeks and, using the same wording as the above study, found prevalence of stress incontinence to be 19% at 8 weeks and 11% by 24 weeks (Thompson et al 2002).

Sleep & Grant (1987a), in following up the population of a trial of perineal management regimes (see guideline on Perineal Pain and Dyspareunia), found a similar prevalence of involuntary loss of urine at the 3-year follow-up (23%) as at the 3-month follow-up (Sleep et al 1984). In a European longitudinal questionnaire-based survey of health problems at 5 and 12 months after birth, 1.7% of women in Italy and 7.6% in France reported urinary incontinence (type not specified) at 5 months. At the 12-month follow-up, this symptom was reported by 5.0% and 14% of women respectively. The prevalences were lower than in other studies, especially in Italy, but in both countries showed an increase over time (Saurel-Cubizolles et al 2000).

Several studies have examined severity or effects on lifestyle of postpartum stress incontinence, with varying findings. Bick & MacArthur (1995), in a questionnaire survey of 1278 women at 6–7 months postpartum, assessed symptom severity using a 100 mm visual analogue scale (VAS), median score being 28 (100 most severe). Although most symptomatic women did not rate stress incontinence as severe, 47% reported wearing pads at some time to protect against their involuntary leakage. Many of the women seemed to view stress incontinence as an expected consequence of childbirth (Bick & MacArthur 1995). In the study by Wilson et al (1996), 129 (25%) of the 516 women with urinary incontinence reported using pads. In the study by Schytt et al (2004) only 2% of the sample had stress incontinence which they considered to be a problem for them. Burgio et al (2003) found that only 6% of women who were symptomatic of incontinence at 12 months felt this restricted their activity at all, although 63% felt that it did disturb them somewhat and 12% felt it disturbed them extremely. In the Canadian study by Hatem et al (2005), two quality of life measures were used and both were found to be significantly worse in the women with urinary incontinence than those without. Dolan et al (2004) measured quality of life using the King's Health Questionnaire and found that among 370 primiparae followed to 3 months postpartum, for 71.1% symptoms had an impact on their life, although for 87.5% of these women this impact was only minor. In a 6-year longitudinal study (MacArthur et al 2006) 12% of symptomatic women had daily or more symptoms and a further 21% had symptoms weekly or more, 23% sometimes and 11% always used a pad to protect against leakage. On a VAS score to assess overall extent of the problem, median score was only 25 but 47% of symptomatic women reported an effect on hygiene, 16% on home life, 35% on social life and 13% on sex life. Mean anxiety and depression scores were also significantly lower in women with incontinence.

## Risk factors

Although childbirth is generally considered to be a major cause of urinary incontinence, and general population studies show it to be more frequent in parous than nulliparous women (Thomas et al 1980, Yarnell et al 1981, 1982, Jolleys 1988, Assassa et al 2000, Hannestad et al 2000, Rortveit et al 2003), the precise causative role of the various factors is still not fully understood.

Urinary incontinence is common during pregnancy and a few cohort studies have followed women and found pregnancy incontinence to be an important risk factor for postpartum incontinence. Schytt et al (2004) found that 21.7% of primiparae and 28.6% of multiparae had involuntary loss of urine in the last trimester of pregnancy; this was found to be a strong predictor of postpartum stress incontinence in both vaginal and caesarean section deliveries. Burgio et al (2003) found that 59.5% of the 523 women in their study experienced involuntary loss of urine at some time during the pregnancy and that this was a strong predictor of postpartum incontinence. Viktrup et al (2006) followed up 241 women 12 years after their first pregnancy. They found that onset during pregnancy as well as onset within the first 3 months was predictive of symptoms at 12 years.

Obstetric factors have been examined in both epidemiological and urodynamic studies. Caesarean section has consistently been found to be associated with less subsequent incontinence (MacArthur et al 1991, Wilson et al 1996, Assassa et al 2000, Hannestad et al 2000, Burgio et al 2003, Schytt et al 2004, Glazener at al 2006, Viktrup 2006). This is consistent with findings of urodynamic investigations of pelvic floor damage (Snooks et al 1986). Even though there is a reduced risk after caesarean section, longitudinal studies have found the prevalence, even in women who only ever delivered operatively, was still about 15% (Hannestad et al 2000, MacArthur et al 2006).

Several urodynamic investigations have found pelvic floor damage to be more common after a longer second-stage labour and the delivery of a bigger baby, but findings relating to forceps delivery have been inconsistent (Snooks et al 1984, 1986, Allen et al 1990, Meyer et al 1998). In the surveys by MacArthur et al (1991) and Brown & Lumley (1998), stress incontinence was found to be more common after forceps delivery and longer second-stage labour. However, the two are closely interrelated and the effect of forceps disappeared (MacArthur et al 1991), or became only marginally significant (Brown & Lumley 1998), after taking duration of second-stage labour into account. Several other large studies have found no association with forceps or instrumental deliveries on multivariate analyses (Farrell et al 2001, MacArthur et al 2001, Schytt et al 2004, Glazener et al 2006), although some smaller studies have found a weak positive association (Viktrup 2002, Burgio et al 2003, Dolan et al 2004). Thompson et al (2002) found an association between stress incontinence and instrumental delivery only at 8 weeks but not at 16 and 24 weeks postpartum.

Older maternal age has been found in numerous studies to be a risk factor for urinary incontinence (MacArthur et al 1991, Fritel et al 2004, Schytt et al 2004, Glazener et al 2006) as well as multiparity (Assassa et al 2000, MacArthur et al 1991, 2006, Schytt et al 2004, Wilson et al 1996). High body mass index (BMI) or obesity (Wilson et al 1996, Burgio et al 2003, Schytt et al 2004, Viktrup et al 2006) as well as heavier infant birthweight (MacArthur et al 1991, Hojberg et al 1999) have also been identified as risk factors in some studies.

## Management

The management of urinary incontinence mainly involves the use of pelvic floor muscle exercises (PFME), either in isolation or combined with some form of biofeedback, although there has been one small trial on the use of weighted vaginal cones. Since the last edition of this book there have been several additional RCTs and systematic reviews investigating the effects of behavioural techniques on urinary incontinence in childbearing women. Some of these have evaluated *antenatal* interventions aimed at *preventing* postpartum incontinence, so are not strictly relevant in a chapter on postnatal management. In the most relevant systematic review, 'Physical therapies for *prevention* of urinary and faecal incontinence in adults', most of the included trials are in childbearing women (Hay-Smith et al 2002). However, this review includes trials with antenatal and postnatal interventions. Another systematic review of pelvic floor exercises, both during and after pregnancy, did not include trials which assessed treatment rather than prevention of urinary incontinence (Harvey 2003). So rather than describe the overall findings of these reviews, we describe here the individual trials in which the intervention to reduce incontinence was delivered postnatally.

Sleep & Grant (1987b) undertook an RCT including 1800 postpartum women of any parity who had had a vaginal delivery. Whilst still in hospital, all women received group-based instruction on pelvic floor exercises from the obstetric physiotherapist, which was standard care. Women in the intervention group also received individual instruction daily whilst in hospital from a midwife co-ordinator. At 3 months postpartum the prevalence of urinary incontinence was similar in both groups (odds ratio (OR) 1.00, 95% confidence interval (CI) 0.83–1.2).

An RCT in Australia included 720 postnatal women who were considered to be at higher risk of urinary incontinence (had instrumental delivery or baby 4000 g+) (Chiarelli & Cockburn 2002). Control was usual care and the intervention was two sessions of individual physiotherapist instruction, one before hospital discharge and the second at 8 weeks postpartum. Significantly fewer women in the intervention group reported urinary incontinence at 12 weeks postpartum relative to controls (OR 0.81, 95% CI 0.66–0.99).

The effects of PFME and bladder training in the treatment of women who were symptomatic of postnatal incontinence at 3 months postpartum (thus not included in the systematic review of prevention) were examined in an RCT in New Zealand (Wilson & Herbison 1998). This trial found significantly less urinary incontinence at 12 months postpartum in the intervention group, but because just over half the women withdrew prior to 12-month assessment relative to only 22% of controls, substantial bias was possible. The intervention was tested again in a much larger multicentre RCT with good follow-up and similar in the treatment and standard care controls (Glazener et al 2001). Symptomatic women (n = 747) were randomly allocated, after stratifying for mode of delivery, frequency of symptoms and parity (para 4 vs 3 or less), to the control (standard postnatal advice) or the intervention group. The intervention was intensive home-based instructions on PFME and bladder retraining from a specially trained midwife or health visitor at 4, 7 and 9 months postpartum. Assessment at 12 months found that significantly fewer of the intervention group were still symptomatic (59.1% vs 69%, diff 9.1%, 95% CI 1.0–19.7%) and significantly more were performing PFME. When these women were followed up at 6 years postpartum, however, there was no difference between groups either in incontinence symptoms or in corresponding PFME practice.

A small non-randomised trial recruited 107 primiparae 2 months after vaginal delivery, some of whom were symptomatic, and randomised them to either 12 one-to-one sessions of pelvic floor re-education with a physiotherapist or standard care. No difference was found between groups in the proportion with urinary incontinence at 10-month postpartum follow-up, but among those who had been symptomatic at recruitment, a significantly higher proportion were 'cured' in the intervention group (Meyer et al 2001).

A non-randomised study of 81 matched pairs comparing intensive postpartum PFME weekly therapy sessions with standard care (Morkved & Bo 2000) found that those who had this therapy programme had significantly less incontinence at 12 months postpartum.

In a systematic review of the effects on urinary incontinence of weighted vaginal cones (Herbison et al 2002), the only trial of childbearing women (Wilson & Herbison 1998) showed no benefit, but this was relatively small and there was substantial and unbalanced drop-out so more evidence on this is needed.

Evidence from RCTs on whether postnatal PFME are effective in managing urinary incontinence therefore is not entirely conclusive, although all but the earliest trial, which had the least intensive therapy, showed positive effects in reducing incontinence up to 12 months postpartum. It is very likely that PMFE will be more effective if performed correctly, and adequate advice and training are necessary to do this (Wilson et al 1987, Bo et al 1988, Bump et al 1991, Morkved & Bo 1996).

## URINARY RETENTION AND VOIDING DIFFICULTIES

Postpartum urinary retention is known to occur but the exact incidence is difficult to ascertain since retention is variably defined and has received little research attention. In a recent review article on postpartum urinary retention, Yip et al (2004) note that a common symptom-based clinical definition is the absence of spontaneous micturition within 6 hours of vaginal delivery and for caeasarean deliveries, no spontaneous micturition within 6 hours after removal of an indwelling catheter (more than 24 hours after delivery). Retention can be covert, being detected by elevated postvoid residual measurements with ultrasound or catheterisation.

In a study of 691 women who had delivered vaginally, Yip et al (1997) found that overall 14.6% had retention on day 1: 9.7% had covert retention, defined as a residual urinary volume of 150 ml or more on day 1, and 4.9% had overt retention, defined as inability to void within 9 hours of delivery because of acute retention. Lee et al (1999), with a definition of residual volume exceeding 200 ml on day 1, found this in 14.1% of 256 vaginal births: 15 women had signs and symptoms and 20 did not. Carley et al (2002) investigated the incidence and factors associated with overt urine retention after vaginal delivery in a retrospective case–control study of 11,332 births and found an incidence of 0.45%. Glavind & Bjork (2003) found an incidence of overt retention of 0.7%, defined as suspicion of retention in the absence of spontaneous micturition within 6 hours of vaginal birth or 6 hours after removal of a catheter in caesarean births, in a hospital sample of 1649 deliveries. Rizvi et al (2005), using the same definition, also found an incidence of 0.7% in a hospital records series in a hospital in Pakistan. Ching-Chung et al (2002), in a study of 2866 vaginal births, found a prevalence of 4% defined as inability to void after delivery and a catheterised bladder volume of >150 ml.

Risk factors for retention, in addition to epidural analgesia (see below), have been found to be instrumental delivery (Lee et al 1999, Ching-Chung et al 2002, Glavind & Bjork 2003) and prolonged labour (Yip et al 1997, Lee et al 1999, Carley et al 2002, Ching-Chung et al 2002).

Epidural analgesia can impede the usual sensory impulses in the bladder, and several studies have found this to be a risk factor for urinary retention (Weil et al 1983, Ramsay and Torbet 1993, Carley et al 2002, Ching-Chung et al 2002). Weil et al (1983), in a urodynamic study of 27 primiparae, found that hypotonic bladders were more common among women delivered vaginally with epidural analgesia, although the study was small. Khullar & Cardozo (1993) studied bladder sensation after epidural and found that it took up to 8 hours for the bladder to regain sensation, within which time more than 1 litre of urine could be produced, which could subsequently damage detrusor function.

Cardozo & Gleeson (1997) have suggested that, in order for overdistension after epidural to be prevented, an indwelling urethral catheter should be inserted at the time of the epidural block and left in situ for 12 hours after the last top-up. Whether ambulatory epidurals, using lower concentrations of anaesthetic agents, have a different effect is not known. More information on the effects of epidural analgesia on the bladder is required.

## Management

There is little research evidence on the management of postpartum urinary retention. It is commonly considered that covert retention is self-limiting. In the study by Yip et al 1997, postresidual bladder volume in women with covert retention spontaneously returned to normal within 4 days. A 4-year follow-up by Yip et al (2002) found the prevalence of subsequent urinary problems of stress incontinence, faecal incontinence, frequency, nocturia, urge incontinence and coital incontinence did not differ in the groups with and without immediate postpartum covert retention. Carley et al (2002) found that 41 of the 51 clinically overt retention cases had resolved by hospital discharge. The remaining 10 were sent home with either intermittent self-catheterisation or indwelling catheter and longest duration of retention was 45 days. Yip et al (2004) note that, although retention may be defined as the absence of spontaneous micturition within 6 hours of a vaginal delivery, the decision to catheterise will depend on the woman's symptoms and physical examination. Basic non-invasive measures, such as providing privacy or having a shower or warm bath, are generally advised first unless symptoms are severe.

## SUMMARY OF THE EVIDENCE USED IN THIS GUIDELINE

- Evidence from numerous large well-conducted observational studies shows that urinary stress incontinence after childbirth is widespread and often persistent. It may have an effect on women's lifestyles, although for most it does not seem to have a major effect.
- Most studies have found the prevalence of urinary incontinence to be lower after caesarean section, but it is still relatively common, even in women who had delivered exclusively by caesarean section. Multiparity and older maternal age are common risk factors. Most studies do not find an association with instrumental delivery.
- Two randomised controlled trials, one non-randomised trial and one matched pair study evaluating PFME-based interventions in the postpartum period indicate a benefit from performing PFME, with less incontinence up to 12 months postpartum. Two trials included only women who were at high risk or symptomatic of incontinence. The trial with negative findings did not make any risk/symptom selection and probably had the least intensive programme.
- Overt and covert retention of urine has been shown in observational studies to be more likely to occur after epidural analgesia, prolonged labour and instrumental delivery. Clinically overt retention is rare. There is little research on management but most cases resolve before hospital discharge.

# WHAT TO DO

## Initial assessment

- Ask about history of present problem.
  - What is the main complaint or symptom and its duration?
- Ask about the following symptoms.
  - Retention/voiding difficulties (such as feeling of incomplete emptying of the bladder; poor stream; straining to void; dysuria; inability to void; awareness of full bladder).
  - Incontinence.
- Ask if the bladder problem interferes with routine activities, or if the woman finds it troublesome in any other way.
- Does the woman need to wear protective pads?

## Conditions which require urgent action

- Retention of urine (expert opinion suggests postvoid residual volume >100 ml).
- Frank incontinence.

## Stress incontinence

- Exclude/detect possible underlying causes: UTI, urinary retention.
- If there is no evidence of a UTI advise normal fluid intake (not more than 2 litres per day).
- Give instructions on how to do pelvic floor muscle exercises, to perform daily.
- If appropriate refer to a continence advisor, e.g. if the woman requires protective pads or finds that the condition interferes with routine tasks (this will be according to local policy; the hospital physiotherapist will be able to advise you on how best to contact him/her if this service is available).
- Reassess symptoms at subsequent visits.
- If condition becomes worse refer to district continence advisor after excluding possible underlying causes.
- If the condition has not improved by the time of final postnatal check advise the woman to tell the GP about this.

## Urinary retention and voiding difficulties

NICE guidelines (NICE 2006) recommend that:

- All women should have their first urine void within 6 hours of giving birth documented in their postnatal record
- If there is no void within 6 hours after birth, active efforts to assist voiding should be advised, such as taking a warm bath or shower
- If a woman has not voided by 6 hours postpartum and measures to encourage micturition are not immediately successful, bladder volume should be assessed and catheterisation considered
- If retention suspected, referral should be made (urgent action).

## How to perform PFME

- Ask the woman what information she has received about PFME and if possible provide any leaflets available from the maternity unit physiotherapy department. Work through the leaflets with her. The following regime is suggested by the Association of Chartered Physiotherapists in Women's Health:-
- Give the mother the following guidance.

*'Squeeze shut the ring of muscle around your back passage (as if stopping a bowel movement), at the same time draw in the muscles around your birth canal (vagina) and LIFT – then relax. Progress to holding the muscles in firmly while you count to FOUR before releasing.*

*Get into a habit of doing these (holding each time for a count of four) after you pass water. If you have difficulty passing water after the birth, it sometimes helps to sit on the toilet and do the pelvic floor exercises with breathing as follows: breathe in as you tighten then sigh the air out as you let go.'*

## SUMMARY GUIDELINE

## Urinary problems

### Initial assessment

- First void within 6 hours of birth should be documented in the postnatal record
- Obtain history of present problem
- Ask about the following symptoms:
  - Incontinence
  - Urgency
  - Voiding difficulties

- Does the problem interfere with routine activities?
- Does the woman need to wear protective pads?

## Urgent action is required if

- Retention of urine
- Frank incontinence

# What to do

### Stress incontinence

- Exclude possible underlying causes such as UTI, retention of urine
- If no evidence of UTI, advise *normal* fluid intake (no more than 2 litres per day)
- Give instructions on pelvic floor muscle exercises to perform daily
- If appropriate, refer to the district continence advisor, e.g. if the woman continues to require protective pads or finds that the condition interferes with routine tasks
- Reassess symptoms at subsequent visits. If condition becomes worse refer to district continence advisor after excluding underlying causes
- If not improved by the final postnatal check, refer (urgent action)

### Urinary retention and voiding difficulties

- If woman has not voided within 6 hours of birth, measures to encourage micturition should be implemented
- Suggest warm bath or shower might assist micturition
- If measures are not immediately successful, bladder volume should be assessed and catheterisation considered
- If retention suspected, refer (urgent action)

### How to perform pelvic floor exercises

Ask the woman what information she has received about PFME, provide leaflets if necessary and work through them with her.

*Squeeze shut the ring of muscle around your back passage (as if stopping a bowel movement), at the same time draw in the muscles around your birth canal (vagina) and LIFT – then relax. Progress to holding the muscles in firmly while you count to FOUR before releasing.*

*Get into a habit of doing these (holding each time for a count of four) after you pass water. If you have difficulty passing water after the birth, it sometimes helps to sit on the toilet and do the pelvic floor exercises with breathing as follows: breathe in as you tighten then sigh the air out as you let go.*

# References

Abrams P, Cardozo L, Fall M et al 2002 Standardisation of terminology of lower urinary tract function: report from the Standardisation Sub-committee of the International Continence Society. Neurourol Urodyn 21: 167-178

Allen R, Hosker G, Smith A 1990 Pelvic floor damage and childbirth: a neurophysiological study. Br J Obstet Gynaecol 97: 770-779

Assassa L, Dallosso S, Perry C et al and the Leicestershire MRC Incontinence Study Team 2000 The association between obstetric factors and incontinence: a community survey. Br J Obstet Gynaecol 107: 822

Bick D, MacArthur C 1995 The extent, severity and effect of health problems after childbirth. Br J Midwif 3: 27-31

Bo K, Larson S, Oseid S et al 1988 Knowledge about and the ability to correct pelvic floor muscle exercises in women with urinary stress incontinence. Neurourol Urodyn 7: 261-262

Brown S, Lumley J 1998 Maternal health after childbirth: results of an Australian population based survey. Br J Obstet Gynaecol 105: 156-161

Bump R, Hurt W, Fantl J et al 1991 Assessment of Kegel pelvic muscle exercise performance after brief verbal instruction. Am J Obstet Gynecol 165(2): 322-329

Burgio K, Matthews K, Engell B 1991 Prevalence, incidence and correlates of urinary incontinence in healthy, middle-aged women. J Urol 146: 1255-1259

Burgio K, Zyczynski H, Locher J et al 2003 Urinary incontinence in the 12-month postpartum period. Obstet Gynecol 102: 1291-1298

Cardozo K, Khullar V 1995 Detrusor instability – drugs and behavioural therapies. In: Smith A (ed.) Urogynaecology. The investigation and management of urinary incontinence in women. RCOG Press, London

Cardozo L, Gleeson C 1997 Pregnancy, childbirth and continence. Br J Midwif 5(5): 277-281

Carley M, Carley J, Vasdev G et al 2002 Factors that are associated with clinically overt postpartum urinary retention after vaginal delivery. Am J Obstet Gynecol 187: 430-433

Chiarelli P, Cockburn J 2002 Promoting urinary continence in women after delivery: randomised controlled trial. BMJ 324: 1241-1246

Ching-Chung L, Shuenn-Dhy C, Ling-Hong T et al 2002 Postpartum urinary retention: assessment of contributing factors and long-term clinical impact. Aust NZ J Obstet Gynaecol 42: 365-368

Dolan L, Walsh D, Hamilton S et al 2004 A study of quality of life in primigravidae with urinary incontinence. Int Urogynecol J 15: 160-164

Farrell S, Allen V, Baskett T 2001 Parturition and urinary incontinence in primiparas. Obstet Gynecol 97: 350-356

Fritel X, Fauconnier A, Levet C et al 2004 Stress urinary incontinence 4 years after the first delivery: a retrospective cohort survey. Acta Obstet Gynecol Scand 83: 941-945

Glavind K, Bjork J 2003 Incidence and treatment of urinary retention postpartum. Int Urogynecol J 14: 119-121

Glazener C, Herbison G, Wilson P et al 2001 Conservative management of persistent postnatal urinary and faecal incontinence: randomised controlled trial. BMJ 323: 593-596

Glazener C, Herbison G, MacArthur C et al 2006 New postnatal urinary incontinence: obstetric and other risk factors in primiparae. Br J Obstet Gynaecol 113: 208-217

Hannestad Y, Rortveit G, Sandvik H et al 2000 A community-based epidemiological survey of female urinary incontinence: the Norwegian EPINCONT study. J Clin Epidemiol 53: 1150-1157

Harvey M-A 2003 Pelvic floor exercises during and after pregnancy: a systematic review of their role in preventing pelvic floor dysfunction. J Obstet Gynaecol Can 56(6): 487-498

Hatem M, Fraser W, Lepire E 2005 Postpartum urinary and anal incontinence: a population-based study of quality of life primiparous women in Quebec. J Obstet Gynaecol Can 27: 682-688

Hay-Smith J, Herbison P, Mordkved S 2002 Physical therapies for prevention of urinary and faecal incontinence in adults. Cochrane Database of Systematic Reviews, Issue 2

Herbison P, Plevnik S, Mantle J 2002 Weighted vaginal cones for urinary incontinence. Cochrane Database of Systematic Reviews, Issue 2

Hojberg K, Salvig J, Winslow N et al 1999 Urinary incontinence: prevalence and risk factors at 16 weeks gestation. Br J Obstet Gynaecol 106: 842-850

Jolleys J 1988 Reported prevalence of urinary incontinence in women in a general practice. BMJ 296: 1300-1302

Khullar V, Cardozo L 1993 Bladder sensation after epidural analgesia. Neurourol Urodyn 12: 424-425

Lee S, Lee C, Tang O et al 1999 Postpartum urinary retention. Int J Gynecol Obstet 66: 287-288

MacArthur C, Lewis M, Knox E 1991 Health after childbirth. HMSO, London

MacArthur C, Glazener CM, Wilson PD et al 2001 Obstetric practice and faecal incontinence three months after delivery. Br J Obstet Gynaecol 108(7): 678-683

MacArthur C, Glazener C, Wilson P et al 2006 Persistent urinary incontinence and delivery mode history: a six-year longitudinal study. Br J Obstet Gynaecol 113: 218-224

Meyer S, Schreyer A, de Grandi P et al 1998 The effects of birth on urinary continence: mechanisms and other pelvic-floor characteristics. Obstet Gynecol 92: 613-618

Meyer S, Hohlfeld P, Achtari C et al 2001 Pelvic floor education after vaginal delivery. Obstet Gynecol 97: 673-677

Morkved S, Bo K 1996 The effect of post-natal exercises to strengthen the pelvic floor muscles. Acta Obstet Gynecol Scand 75: 382-385

Morkved S, Bo K 2000 Effect of postpartum pelvic floor muscle training in prevention and treatment of urinary incontinence: a one-year follow up. Br J Obstet Gynaecol 107: 1022-1028

National Institute for Health and Clinical Excellence (NICE) 2006 Routine postnatal care of women and their babies. Postnatal Care: NICE Clinical Guideline 37

O'Brien J, Austin M, Sethi P et al 1991 Urinary incontinence: prevalence, need for treatment, and effectiveness of intervention by nurse. BMJ 303: 1308-1312

Ramsay I, Torbet T 1993 Incidence of abnormal voiding parameters in the immediate postpartum period. Neurourol Urodyn 12(2): 179-183

Rizvi R, Khan Z, Khan Z 2005 Diagnosis and management of postpartum urinary retention. Int J Gynecol Obstet 91: 71-72

Rortveit G, Daltveit A, Hannestad Y et al 2003 Urinary incontinence after vaginal delivery or cesarean section. N Engl J Med 348: 900-907

Saurel-Cubizolles M-J, Romito P, Lelong N et al 2000 Women's health after childbirth: a longitudinal study in France and Italy. Br J Obstet Gynaecol 107: 1202-1209

Schytt et al E, Lindmark G, Waldenstrom U 2004 Symptoms of stress incontinence 1 year after childbirth: prevalence and predictors in a national Swedish sample. Acta Obstet Gynecol Scand 83: 928-936

Sleep J, Grant A 1987a West Berkshire perineal management trial: three year follow-up. BMJ 295: 749-751

Sleep J, Grant A 1987b Pelvic floor exercises in postnatal care. Midwifery 3: 158-164

Sleep J, Grant A, Garcia J et al 1984 West Berkshire perineal management trial. BMJ 289: 587-590

Snooks S, Setchell M, Swash M et al 1984 Injury to the innervation of pelvic floor sphincter musculature in childbirth. Lancet II: 546-550

Snooks S, Swash M, Henry M et al 1986 Risk factors in childbirth causing damage to the pelvic floor innervation. Int J Colorectal Dis 1: 20-24

Thomas T, Plymat K, Blannin J et al 1980 Prevalence of urinary incontinence. BMJ 281: 1243-1245

Thompson J, Roberts C, Currie M et al 2002 Prevalence and persistence of health problems after childbirth: associations with parity and method of birth. Birth 29: 83-94

Viktrup L 2002 The risk of lower urinary tract symptoms five years after the first delivery. Neurourol Urodyn 21: 2-29

Viktrup L, Rortveit G, Lose G 2006 Risk of stress urinary incontinence twelve years after the first pregnancy and delivery. Obstet Gynecol 108: 248-254

Weil A, Reyes H, Rottenberg R et al 1983 Effect of lumbar epidural analgesia on lower urinary tract function in the immediate postpartum period. Br J Obstet Gynaecol 90: 428-432

Wilson P, Herbison G 1998 A randomised controlled trial of pelvic floor muscle exercises to treat postnatal urinary incontinence. Int Urogynecol J 9: 257-264

Wilson P, Samarrai T, Deakin M et al 1987 An objective assessment of physiotherapy for female genuine stress incontinence. Br J Obstet Gynaecol 94: 575-582

Wilson P, Herbison R, Herbison G 1996 Obstetric practice and the prevalence of urinary incontinence three months after delivery. Br J Obstet Gynaecol 103: 154-161

Yarnell J, Voyle G, Richards C et al 1981 The prevalence and severity of urinary incontinence in women. J Epidemiol Commun Health 35: 71-74

Yarnell J, Voyle G, Sweetnam P et al 1982 Factors associated with urinary incontinence in women. J Epidemiol Commun Health 36: 58-63

Yip S-K, Brieger G, Hin L-Y et al 1997 Urinary retention in the post-partum period. The relationship between obstetric factors and the post-partum post-void residual bladder volume. Acta Obstet Gynecol Scand 76: 667-672

Yip S-K, Sahota D, Chang A et al 2002 Four-year follow-up of women who were diagnosed to have postpartum urinary retention. Am J Obstet Gynecol 187: 648-652

Yip S-K, Sahota D, Pang M-W et al 2004 Postpartum urinary retention. Acta Obstet Gynecol Scand 83: 881-891

## Chapter 6

# Bowel problems

## INTRODUCTION

There are various bowel problems that women can experience following childbirth. Constipation and haemorrhoids have long been known as common postpartum symptoms, and more recent studies have shown that women may also experience faecal incontinence in the postpartum period.

## CONSTIPATION

### Definition

Constipation is defined as difficulty in evacuating the bowel and is a common symptom during the second and third trimesters of pregnancy, arising from relaxation of the smooth muscle of the intestine as a result of circulating progesterone (Shepherd 2004). During the immediate postpartum period women may experience constipation following lack of dietary intake during labour or because of pain from perineal trauma.

### Frequency of occurrence and risk factors

Although it is generally 'well known' that constipation can occur after childbirth, there is little documentary evidence of its prevalence or risk factors. Garcia & Marchant (1993), as part of an in-depth descriptive survey of postnatal care, sent 100 women a postal questionnaire at 8 weeks postpartum to ask about health problems; 90 women responded, 20 (22%) of whom had experienced constipation since their delivery, although onset and duration were not given. In a prospective observational study in Scotland, a representative sample of over 1200 women was surveyed whilst still in hospital, at 8 weeks and at 12–18 months, when half the sample was followed to ask about symptoms after 8 weeks: 19%, 20% and 7% respectively reported constipation at these various times (Glazener et al 1995). In a longitudinal survey by Saurel-Cubizolles et al (2000), 13% of the Italian women and 14% of the French reported constipation at 5 months. At 12 months these proportions were 17% and 26% respectively.

At all survey periods in the study by Glazener et al (1995), univariate analysis showed that constipation was significantly more common among women following instrumental deliveries, compared with spontaneous vaginal deliveries or caesarean sections. The proportions reporting constipation were, respectively, 31%, 17% and 20% in hospital, 31%, 18% and 17% between then and 8 weeks, and 14%, 6% and 5% after this. Constipation whilst still in hospital was found to be more common among primiparae (23%) than multiparae (16%), but after this the parity difference was nonsignificant (Glazener et al 1995). Since primiparae have much higher rates of instrumental deliveries than multiparae, the parity association may not be an independent one.

Schytt et al (2004) asked about constipation in a longitudinal study investigating urinary stress incontinence and found a prevalence of 21.7% and 28.6% in the third trimester among primiparae and multiparae respectively; these proportions were 25% and 29.3% at 4–8 weeks postpartum and 22% and 25.6% at 1 year. Constipation at 4–8 weeks was a significant independent predictor of stress incontinence at 1 year postpartum. French women who reported constipation at 12 months in the survey by Saurel-Cubizolles et al (2000) were more likely to be in employment, but there was no similar difference among the Italian women.

A longitudinal study in The Netherlands of 407 women, followed at 3 and 12 months postpartum to investigate defaecatory symptoms during and after a first pregnancy, found a much lower prevalence of constipation at 4.6% and 4.2% respectively but the definition (less than three bowel movements a week and need to strain 25% or more of the time) was more restrictive than in other studies. Independent risk factors for this were constipation at 12 weeks gestation and higher body mass index (BMI) (van Brummen et al 2006).

## Management

There is limited research into the most effective treatment of constipation among either obstetric or non-obstetric populations and most conservative management of postpartum constipation is based on current clinical practice.

Jewell & Young (2001), in a Cochrane systematic review of interventions for the treatment of constipation during pregnancy, found two trials. One trial including 40 women showed that bran and wheat supplements were effective in increasing the frequency of defaecation (odds ratio (OR) 0.18, 95% confidence interval (CI) 0.05–0.67) and unlikely to have side-effects for the mother or fetus. The other trial, reporting on 140 women, found that stimulant laxatives were more effective than bulk-forming laxatives (OR 0.30, 95% CI 0.14–0.61) but may cause side-effects.

In an early randomised controlled trial in South Africa, comparing the use of the laxative senna (n = 224) with placebo (n = 247) for immediate postpartum constipation, senna was shown to be effective in producing spontaneous bowel action, but 12% of cases compared with 3% of controls experienced abdominal cramps, although most were described as mild (Shelton 1980).

Tramonte et al (1997) undertook a systematic review of general population trials (peripartum trials excluded) to evaluate whether laxatives and fibre therapy, for a minimum of 1 week, improved symptoms in adults who had experienced constipation for at least 2 weeks. Thirty six trials were included, with a total of 1815 subjects and a range of different laxative and fibre treatments. The reviewers concluded that both fibre and laxatives modestly improved bowel movement frequency but there was insufficient evidence to determine whether fibre was superior to laxative treatment or whether one class of laxative was better than another. They suggested that laxatives should only be given when simple treatments, such as fibre and dietary interventions, have failed.

## HAEMORRHOIDS

### Definition

Haemorrhoids result from swollen veins around the anus, which in severe cases can prolapse. Haemorrhoids can be graded according to the degree of prolapse: first-degree haemorrhoids are visible but do not prolapse; second-degree haemorrhoids prolapse with defaecation but return spontaneously; third-degree haemorrhoids prolapse and require manual replacement; and fourth-degree haemorrhoids remain prolapsed outside the anal canal (Pfenninger 1997). Haemorrhoids may occur during pregnancy as a result of the action of progesterone on the bowel, which increases varicosity, and during the postnatal period possibly as a consequence of pushing in the second stage of labour.

### Frequency of occurrence and risk factors

Like constipation, haemorrhoids are considered to be a 'well-known' consequence of childbirth. Midwifery and obstetric textbooks have generally noted that haemorrhoids can cause a great deal of pain for a few days after delivery but then resolve, although they may worsen with subsequent pregnancies and can eventually become permanent (Hibbard 1988). More recently, however, observational studies of health problems after childbirth have found that haemorrhoids, whether of pregnancy or postpartum onset, do not always resolve quickly. MacArthur et al (1991), in an observational study, found that among 11,701 women 8% reported haemorrhoids of more than 6 weeks' duration starting for the first time within 3 months of birth, and an additional 10% had ongoing or recurrent symptoms. Two-thirds of symptomatic women still had haemorrhoids at questioning, 1–9 years after delivery. Multivariate analysis showed that new symptoms were independently associated with forceps delivery, longer second-stage labour and vaginal delivery of a heavier baby. They were less likely after caesarean section and if delivered by section, there was no association with birthweight. These associations are all compatible with a longer or more expulsive period of pushing.

Glazener et al (1995), in a longitudinal study, found that 17% of women reported haemorrhoids (new and recurrent) when questioned in hospital, 22% between then and 8 weeks and 15% after this. As in the study by MacArthur et al (1991), haemorrhoids were significantly more common with an instrumental than a spontaneous vaginal delivery, and significantly less common with a caesarean section: 27%, 17% and 6% respectively whilst in hospital; and 31%, 23% and 14% between then and 8 weeks. At 12–18 months, however, no difference was found in haemorrhoids after 8 weeks in the spontaneous vaginal delivery (SVD) group (13%) relative to the caesarean section group (11%), but there were still significantly more in the instrumental delivery group (30%). Relationships with other factors, such as duration of second-stage labour or birthweight, were not reported.

Brown & Lumley (1998), in a population-based Australian survey at 6–7 months postpartum, found that haemorrhoids that women considered to be a problem for them were significantly associated with mode of delivery, occurring after 36% of instrumental deliveries, 25% of spontaneous vaginal deliveries, 17% of elective and 11% of emergency sections. Thompson et al (2002), in a longitudinal study in Australia, using similar questioning to Brown & Lumley (1998), found that the prevalence of haemorrhoids reduced over the first 6 months after birth from 30% between 0 and 8 weeks, to 18% at 16 weeks, but prevalence was still 13% between 16 and 24 weeks. Haemorrhoids were proportionately more common among women who had assisted compared with spontaneous vaginal deliveries and less common among those who had caesarean births, but these differences were not statistically significant. Ansara et al (2005), in a Canadian study, again using similar questioning to Brown & Lumley (1998), found the prevalence of haemorrhoids at 8–10 weeks postpartum to be 35.5%. After adjusting for several factors, including episiotomy and duration of labour, they found an independent positive association between haemorrhoids and instrumental relative to a spontaneous delivery (OR 2.57, 95% CI 1.16–5.70) and a negative association for caesarean section (OR 0.36, 95% CI 0.16–0.81).

In a European longitudinal study (Saurel-Cubizolles et al 2000) the prevalence of haemorrhoids among French and Italian women at 5 months postpartum was 16% in both cases, and prevalence at 12 months had increased to 21% among Italian and 26% among the French women. The authors suggest various reasons for this increase in symptoms, including a change in women's perception of their health, so symptoms by then may feel more bothersome, as well as the effect of increasing demands of the baby.

## Management

Treatment options available for haemorrhoids are varied and generally depend on severity, with scalpel surgery now reserved only for advanced fourth-degree cases (Pfenninger 1997).

Only one systematic review has been found specifically concerning post-partum populations. This review, published in 2005, is of 'conservative management of symptomatic and/or complicated haemorrhoids in pregnancy and the puerperium' (Quijano & Abalos 2005). Only two RCTs were found in childbearing populations, both of which were comparing phlebotonics (oral rutosides) with placebo during pregnancy, with no trials in postpartum populations. The authors concluded that, although this form of treatment looked promising for symptom relief in first- and second-degree haemorrhoids, its use cannot be recommended until new evidence provides reassurances about safety.

Like constipation, the conservative management of less severe childbirth-related haemorrhoids is based on current clinical practice. Relief of mild haemorrhoids may be provided by the topical application of creams, and dietary advice to ensure avoidance of constipation is also usually given, but there is no trial evidence of their effectiveness in either pregnant or postpartum populations. Alonso-Coello et al (2006) have recently completed a Cochrane review of laxatives for the treatment of haemorrhoids. This review found seven RCTs with a total of 378 participants, all in general populations, and concluded that laxatives in the form of fibre had a beneficial effect in the treatment of symptomatic haemorrhoids; the risk of not improving haemorrhoids and having persistent symptoms decreased by 53% in the fibre group (RR 0.47, 95% CI 0.32–0.68).

If haemorrhoids are severe and further treatment is required there are now numerous options, including rubber band ligation, cryothermy, injection sclerotherapy, infrared coagulation, diathermy and operative haemorrhoidectomy (MacRae & MacLeod 1995, Pfenninger 1997). No trials have specifically evaluated treatments for severe haemorrhoids in the postpartum period.

## FAECAL INCONTINENCE

### Definition

Faecal incontinence refers to the involuntary passage of bowel contents. The term is usually used to refer to solid or liquid faeces, which can be frank incontinence or soiling or staining of underwear, although faecal urgency is often also included. Faecal urgency is where the sensation of needing a bowel movement is felt but defaecation can only be deferred for a short period (a limit of 5 minutes or less is often given). Sometimes flatus incontinence is also included, although anal incontinence seems a more appropriate term used to refer to incontinence of faeces and/or flatus. There is currently no standard definition or classificatory system and no standard form of questioning, so differences in estimates of incidence and prevalence of faecal incontinence will occur. Where possible, the definition and method of ascertainment are described for each study.

## Frequency of occurrence

It has long been recognised that childbirth is important in the pathogenesis of faecal incontinence based on histories of middle-aged women presenting in colorectal clinics, but until studies in the 1990s showed otherwise, it was generally assumed that women rarely (except after a third-degree tear) became symptomatic in the postpartum period (Swash 1993). In addition to epidemiological studies investigating prevalence and risk factors of faecal incontinence, there are data on symptom occurrence from pathophysiological studies of occult anal sphincter injury, and from studies primarily examining other problems (usually urinary incontinence). Since the last edition of this book, there has been a substantial increase in the number of studies on this topic.

### Epidemiological studies

Sleep & Grant (1987), in a large randomised controlled trial of the effectiveness of pelvic floor exercises on urinary incontinence at 3 months postpartum, reported as an incidental finding that 3% of the women in the intervention and control groups experienced 'occasional faecal loss' but this was not mentioned further. Wilson et al (1996), in a study in New Zealand on the prevalence of urinary incontinence at 3 months postpartum, asked about faecal incontinence (new and recurrent symptoms, not including flatus) and found that 73 of the 1505 women (4.9%) experienced this, although they reported no further details.

An observational study in Birmingham, UK, of several health problems, including faecal incontinence, at 10 months postpartum obtained information on the incidence, duration and nature of this in a representative sample of 906 women (MacArthur et al 1997). Research midwives, in home-based interviews, asked about frank incontinence, soiling or staining of underwear, or urgency (described as 'felt the need to go but couldn't hold on'). Of the 906 women, 36 (4%) had experienced one or more of these as a new postpartum problem, the majority reporting onset as immediate or in the first 2 weeks. A further 19 women (2%) had recurrent or ongoing symptoms from a previous birth (n = 7) or because of a pre-existing condition (n = 12), mostly irritable bowel syndrome. Mean symptom duration among the 36 with new symptoms was 23 weeks; only five women had consulted their GP and 14 (39%) cases had resolved by the time of interview.

Zetterström et al (1999), in a prospective study in Sweden of anal inconti-nence among 278 primiparae who had a vaginal birth , found a low symp-tom frequency. At 5 months postpartum, five women (1.8%) reported incontinence of faeces and 70 (25%) of flatus, and at 9 months only three (1.1%) reported faecal and 71 (25%) flatus incontinence. A cross-sectional study from Israel (Groutz et al 1999) also found a low symptom frequency among 300 women interviewed at 3 months postpartum: 21 (7%) reported anal incontinence, two of faeces (0.7%), the remainder of flatus (6.3%). None had sought medical consultation. The European longitudinal survey of women's health after childbirth found faecal incontinence rates at 5 months of 1% of 697 women in Italy and 3% of 589 women in France, and 3% and 5% respectively at 12 months (Saurel-Cubizolles et al 2000). Symptoms were self-reported with no definition of faecal incontinence given.

As part of a randomised controlled trial of treatment for postpartum uri-nary incontinence in high-risk women (instrumental births and baby 4000 g+) in Australia, data on faecal incontinence were also collected from the 568 women who were followed up at 12 months (Chiarelli et al 2003). Prev-alence of faecal incontinence (ever accidentally lose solid or liquid stool) was 6.9%, 2.6% and 4.9% respectively, including some women with both. A mul-ticentre study in England, Scotland and New Zealand also collected data on faecal incontinence from the whole study cohort (MacArthur et al 2001), whilst recruiting and following women as part of an RCT of treatment for urinary incontinence (Glazener et al 2001). At 3 months postpartum 7879 questionnaires were returned (72% response rate) and the prevalence of fae-cal incontinence (ever lose control of bowel motions from back passage in between visits to the toilet) was 9.6%. Six years after this birth the women were followed again, when 4214 responded. Of these, a total of 10% had fae-cal incontinence at that time; 3.6% had faecal incontinence on both occasions (MacArthur et al 2005). There was substantial resolution of symptoms and appearance of new ones: in 59% of the women who had symptoms at 3 months these had resolved, and 64% of women had symptoms at 6 years that had not been present at 3 months.

Several other recent studies have investigated postpartum faecal inconti-nence, with varying prevalence estimates. In a French study of 159 women who had instrumental deliveries and excluding women with previous anal incontinence, prevalence of loss of liquid or solid stool was 8.8% (Mazouni et al 2005). In a longitudinal study of 242 women up to 5 years following first delivery (excluding caesarean sections), prevalence of incontinence to solid or loose stool was 1% at 9 months and 5.4% at 5 years (Pollack et al 2004). A longitudinal study of 407 women followed at 3 and 12 months after birth in The Netherlands found prevalence of incontinence to liquid or solid stool to be 5.7% and 3.3% respectively (van Brummen et al 2006).

## Pathophysiological studies

Investigative techniques developed in the 1990s, in particular endosonogra-phy and manometry, have enabled imaging of the anal sphincter muscles, and several studies of occult damage to internal or external anal sphincters have been undertaken. Most of these also obtained symptom data, but generally found higher symptom prevalences than in the epidemiological studies, probably because consent to the various anal investigations is more likely in symptomatic women. One study has demonstrated this (Chaliha et al 2001).

The first of these types of studies was undertaken by Sultan and colleagues (1993), who carried out examinations on 202 women who agreed to take part at 34 weeks' gestation, and 150 who returned for further investigations at 6–8 weeks postpartum. Each time, the women completed a symptom questionnaire, which recorded anal incontinence, including faecal and flatus incontinence, and faecal urgency (defined as inability to defer defaecation for more than 5 minutes). Among the 150 women followed, 21 (14%) reported postpartum bowel control symptoms, 13 (8.7%) had new symptoms and eight (5.3%) recurrent or ongoing ones. Anal endosonography among the 79 primiparae who had delivered vaginally showed that none of these women had occult sphincter defects antenatally, but at 6–8 weeks 28 (35%) had defects. Among the multiparae 19 (40%) had defects antenatally and 22 (44%) at postnatal follow-up. The fact that postpartum incidence of defects among the primiparae was similar to the antenatal incidence of defects among multiparae indicates that anal sphincter damage is most likely following the first delivery. All except one of the women with anal incontinence or faecal urgency had a sphincter defect. Sphincter defects, however, were more common than symptoms; only about one-third of the women with defects experienced any loss of bowel control.

Similar studies followed that by Sultan et al and a meta-analysis to determine the incidence of obstetric anal sphincter damage and associated incidences of faecal incontinence was published in 2003 (Oberwalder et al 2003). It identified five studies published up to July 2001, including the one by Sultan et al (1993) described above. Based on a total of 717 vaginal deliveries, the incidence of anal sphincter defect in primiparae was found to be 26.9% and the incidence of new defects in multiparae was 8.5%. Overall, 29.7% of all women with defects were symptomatic (varying symptom definitions) and 3–4% of women experienced symptoms without a defect.

A large study, published since this meta-analysis, included 286 nulliparous women who underwent anorectal sensation and manometric examinations and completed a symptom questionnaire in the third trimester of pregnancy (Chaliha et al 2001). One hundred and sixty one women returned for the anorectal investigations and questionnaire completion at 3 months postpartum and the remaining 125 women completed the questionnaire by telephone. Overall prevalence of anal incontinence (including flatus) at 3 months was 10.5% and was 8.7%. for faecal urgency. Symptom prevalence was significantly greater in the women who returned for investigations.

## Risk factors

Epidemiological and pathophysiological studies are generally in agreement that the two main factors associated with the occurrence of faecal incontinence and with occult anal sphincter defects are instrumental delivery and third-/fourth-degree tear.

In an early epidemiological study of 906 women by MacArthur et al (1997), obstetric data from case notes were obtained, and logistic regression showed that forceps and vacuum extraction delivery were the only maternal or obstetric factors that were independently associated with new faecal incontinence reported by the women. Zetterström et al (1999), in Sweden, found a relationship between instrumental delivery and anal incontinence at 5 months postpartum, but not at 9 months. This was a small study, however, and the authors noted that the 10% instrumental delivery rate among the primiparous sample was very low and may have affected these findings. Groutz et al (1999) also found a relationship between anal incontinence and instrumental delivery, although again the small sample size makes information on risk factors highly tentative. Moreover, almost all of the instrumental deliveries in both these studies were by vacuum extraction. A community-based general population study of over 6000 women (median age 58 years) showed that having ever had a forceps birth was significantly associated with faecal incontinence (OR 1.5), although how long after the birth the symptoms had begun was not available (Assassa et al 2000).

In the study of occult sphincter damage by Sultan et al (1993), the only obstetric factor independently associated with damage was forceps delivery: eight of the 10 women delivered by forceps had sphincter defects, although none of five delivered by vacuum extraction had defects. Donnelly et al (1998), in their Dublin study of sphincter damage in 124 primiparous women, found that instrumental delivery was associated with an 8.1-fold (95% CI 2.7–24.0) risk of anal sphincter injury and a 7.2-fold (95% CI 2.8–18.6) risk of symptoms (urgency, faecal and flatus incontinence). Abramowitz et al (2000), included in the earlier meta-analysis of anal sphincter damage, found forceps delivery to be an independent predictor of damage (OR 12, 95% CI 4–20).

Most studies are too small to allow a definite conclusion about the relative effects of instrumental delivery by forceps or by vacuum extraction. MacArthur et al (2001), in a large study of 4214 women at 3 months postpartum, were able to separately examine associations with each of the instruments. This showed that relative to spontaneous vaginal delivery, forceps delivery was independently associated with faecal incontinence (OR 1.94, 95% CI 1.29–1.30), but vacuum extraction was not (OR 1.26, 95% CI 0.77–2.07). A small trial randomised women who required an instrumental delivery to forceps (n = 61) or vacuum extraction (n = 69) and found that a significantly greater proportion of women in the forceps group reported altered faecal continence but no significant difference in continence score or faecal urgency was found (Fitzpatrick et al 2003). A small case–control study of 50 vacuum extraction and 50 spontaneous vaginal deliveries, matched for perineal trauma, showed that anal incontinence rates (urgency, flatus, liquid stool and soiling) were the same in both groups (Peschers et al 2003).

Third-degree tears have long been known to increase the risk of subsequent faecal incontinence but this type of trauma, as recorded in case notes, is uncommon, occurring in 0.5–1% of vaginal deliveries (Kamm 1998). In a study of a UK hospital population of 8603 vaginal deliveries, 50 (0.6%) were recorded as having third-degree tear (Sultan et al 1994). Thirty four of the 50 women with this trauma agreed to be further investigated and were matched for parity, age and ethnic origin with 88 controls, none of whom had ever had a third-degree tear. Anal incontinence (including flatus) or faecal urgency was present in 16 women (42%) with tears and 11 controls (13%). A US study of the incidence and outcome of third-degree tear among 16,853 vaginal deliveries found 93 (0.5%) recorded cases; 81 of these were reviewed 3 months after, at which time 16 (20%) suffered from anal incontinence (including flatus) (Walsh et al 1996). A similar study in Adelaide, Australia, of 9613 vaginal deliveries identified 116 (1.2%) third-degree tears (Wood et al 1998). Eighty four of these were interviewed by telephone, 14 (17%) of whom had faecal or flatus incontinence and seven had other symptoms of anal dysfunction. Most epidemiological studies of faecal incontinence have not investigated third-degree tear as a risk factor because of small numbers. Van Brummen et al (2006) and Pollack et al (2004) did examine this and found third-degree tear to be an independent predictor of faecal incontinence.

Perineal laceration (excluding third-degree tear) has not been found to be associated with either faecal incontinence symptoms or occult anal sphincter damage (Chiarelli et al 2003, MacArthur et al 1997, 2001, van Brummen et al 2006). Most studies do not find an association either with episiotomy but there are exceptions. Signorello et al (2000), in a retrospective cohort study in the USA, examined the effects of midline episiotomy, questioning equal numbers of women with episiotomy (n = 205), tear (n = 204) and intact perineum (n = 203). At 3 months postpartum the prevalence of faecal incontinence was 2.4% in the intact group, 3.4% after tear and 9.9% after episiotomy. At 6 months the retrospective proportions were 1.5%, 1.5% and 4.3%, indicating a significant excess in the episiotomy group on both occasions. This type of episiotomy, midline, is rarely used in the UK and the retrospective cohort study design, with substantial potential for bias, renders findings inconclusive. Groutz et al (1999) found an association but this was not independent of instrumental delivery because almost all were accompanied by episiotomy. A recent study by Andrews et al (2006), including 241 women having a first vaginal delivery of whom 59 sustained anal sphincter injuries, found that mediolateral episiotomy was an independent risk factor for these injuries (OR 4.04, 95% CI 1.71–9.56). Episiotomies angled closer to the midline were more likely to incur injury.

Several other independent risk factors of faecal incontinence have been found, but not all consistently so. Older maternal age was positively associated with faecal incontinence at 3 months and at 6 years in the study by MacArthur et al (2001, 2005), and with anal incontinence at 5 months and 9 months postpartum in the Swedish study (Zetterström et al 1999), but not with anal incontinence at 12 months in the Australian study (Chiarelli et al 2003). Epidural analgesia was found to be independently associated with bowel control symptoms and with anal sphincter damage by Donnelly et al (1998) in their Dublin study, although Zetterström et al (1999), van Brummen et al (2006) and Sartore et al (2003) in their studies found no relationship. Yao et al (2006) found multiparity to be a risk factor for faecal incontinence. MacArthur et al (2001) found a clear trend for two, three and four or more births relative to one, and Chiarelli et al (2003) found an independent association for multiparity relative to primiparity. MacArthur et al (2001, 2005) found an independent positive association between faecal incontinence and Asian ethnic group, but no other studies have been found that have investigated this.

There has been much discussion about whether caesarean section delivery is *protective* against subsequent faecal incontinence (Sultan & Stanton 1996) and this has been used as 'evidence' by informed women to request an elective caesarean section (Al-Mufti et al 1997). MacArthur et al (1997) in their first study found six reports of new faecal incontinence symptoms following 113 emergency sections and none following 61 elective sections, the rate of the former being similar to that following spontaneous vaginal delivery. In a much larger subsequent study, they found that symptoms 3 months after birth were marginally less likely among the primiparous women who had a caesarean section (OR 0.58, 95% CI 0.35–0.97) (MacArthur et al 2001). However, when followed up at 6 years, at which time information on mode of all deliveries of the women had been obtained, it was shown clearly that delivering, even exclusively, by caesarean section was not associated with fewer symptoms (OR 1.04, 95% CI 0.72–1.50). Looking separately at 116 women who only ever delivered by *caesarean section before labour*, 16 were symptomatic at 6 years compared with 22 of the 300 who had one or more sections after the onset of labour, which does not seem to support the earlier suppositions that even elective sections are predictive of fewer symptoms (MacArthur et al 2005).

The pathophysiological study by Sultan et al (1993) found that none of seven women delivered by elective section, nor the 16 delivered by emergency section, had anal or bowel symptoms or sphincter defects, but there was evidence of pudendal nerve neuropathy among the emergency section group. Fynes et al (1998) studied 34 primiparous women, of whom eight had elective section before labour, 17 had emergency section before 8 cm dilatation and nine had emergency section after 8 cm dilatation; the authors found that none reported alteration in bowel function at 6 weeks, nor was there any evidence of mechanical anal sphincter damage, irrespective of when the section had been performed. Those who delivered in late labour, however, even without attempted vaginal delivery, had signs of pudendal nerve damage, which is compatible with the findings of Sultan et al (1993).

Pathophysiological studies, although based on small numbers of caesarean deliveries, seem to show little evidence of mechanical anal sphincter damage after caesarean section, but that damage to the innervation of the anal sphincter can still occur. The large epidemiological studies show no reduction in faecal incontinence even in women who only ever delivered abdominally. Since the searches for this book were completed, a newly published systematic review has been published, confirming this conclusion (Nelson et al 2006). This review of the 'efficacy of caesarean section in the preservation of anal incontinence' found 15 studies encompassing 3010 caesarean sections and 11,440 vaginal births which reported data on faecal incontinence. The summary relative risk from these studies for faecal incontinence following caesarean section was 0.91 (95% CI 0.74–1.14) and was 0.98 (95% CI 0.86–1.13) for incontinence of flatus. The conclusion of this review was that caesarean section does not prevent anal incontinence. On balance, therefore, the current evidence does not seem to support caesarean section being associated with a reduced likelihood of subsequent faecal incontinence.

## Management

Faecal incontinence as an immediate consequence of childbirth, even without anal sphincter rupture, is clearly more common than previously suspected, and since few women spontaneously report its occurrence, it is important that midwives specifically ask about bowel control symptoms as part of delivering postnatal care. It has been suggested that women with persistent symptoms of loss of bowel control should be reviewed by a colorectal specialist, but this decision will depend on local policy (Cook & Mortensen 1998).

Treatment options for non-transient faecal incontinence include conservative therapies as well as surgery. Conservative therapy consists of regulating the stool form using a high-fibre diet and antidiarrhoeal agents, and pelvic floor exercises, with or without biofeedback, but there is insufficient evidence on effectiveness of these. One trial investigating pelvic floor muscle exercises (PFME) as a treatment in women symptomatic of urinary incontinence at 3 months postpartum also assessed faecal incontinence at 12 months and found these symptoms to be significantly reduced in the PFME group relative to controls (Glazener et al 2001). At 6 years, however, there were no symptom differences (Glazener et al 2005). Women with faecal incontinence in this trial were only included if also symptomatic of urinary incontinence, so although it was a large trial, there were only 57 women in the intervention group and 54 controls with faecal incontinence at baseline. More research on this is needed.

There have been two randomised controlled trials undertaken by a team in Dublin examining the effects of various forms of intra-anal electromyographic biofeedback, one in women who had impaired faecal continence after anal sphincter tear (Fynes et al 1999) and the other in any women symptomatic at 12 weeks postpartum (Mahony et al 2004). These have shown that these types of treatment were associated with improved continence. However, the trials were small (n = 36 and 52 respectively) and did not compare the treatments with standard pelvic floor exercise techniques. Larger randomised controlled trials are needed.

There is concern about whether third-degree tears are correctly identified by doctors and midwives, so that some remain unrecorded, and about the inadequate knowledge of their repair (Sultan et al 1995). A recent randomised controlled trial of 752 primiparous women without a clinically evident anal sphincter tear investigated the effect of adding endoanal ultrasound immediately after vaginal delivery, with diagnosed tears then surgically explored and sutured (Faltin et al 2005). Severe faecal incontinence was significantly reduced at 3 months postpartum relative to the standard care control group (3.3% vs 8.7%, diff. −5.4%, 95% CI −8.9 to −2.0).

A recent Cochrane review of methods of repair for obstetric anal sphincter injury (Fernando et al 2006) found three trials involving 279 women comparing overlap versus end-to-end repair. The results show that early primary overlap repair appeared to be associated with lower risks of faecal urgency and anal incontinence, but these conclusions are tentative, also because the experience of the surgeons in the techniques was not adequately addressed. In terms of conservative management of third-degree tear, expert opinion suggests that women should be prescribed prophylactic laxatives for 2 weeks to prevent constipation. However, prospective studies are required to establish the most appropriate management of such women.

## SUMMARY OF THE EVIDENCE USED IN THIS GUIDELINE

- Numerous observational studies have now indicated that all the postnatal bowel symptoms described in this guideline are relatively common. Most occur within the first week or two after delivery and all have been shown sometimes to persist.
- Conservative treatment of postpartum constipation and haemorrhoids is largely based on current general population clinical practice.
- Various types of observational studies have clearly demonstrated that faecal incontinence symptoms, occult anal sphincter damage and third-degree tears are more common after instrumental deliveries.
- Pathophysiological studies have demonstrated that occult anal sphincter damage occurs after about a third of first vaginal births and rarely after this. Bowel control symptoms are much less common than defects but if a defect occurs, symptoms after subsequent vaginal deliveries are more likely.

- One large longitudinal study has shown that delivering exclusively by caesarean section does not significantly reduce the risk of faecal incontinence. Pathophysiological studies indicate that although mechanical anal sphincter damage does not seem to occur after caesarean section, neurological damage can occur.
- There is consensus that third-degree tear confers an increased risk of faecal incontinence, but since these tears are relatively rare, most women with faecal incontinence will not have had this type of trauma.
- More good-quality studies are needed on the management of women with postpartum faecal incontinence.
- There is consensus that women do not spontaneously report bowel control symptoms but if asked (as shown in studies), will disclose this symptomatology.

## WHAT TO DO

### Initial assessment

- Ask if bowels opened since giving birth. NICE (2006) recommends that women are asked about this within 3 days of the birth.
- Ask about specific difficulties to enable identification of the following – constipation, haemorrhoids, loss of bowel control, including soiling, faecal urgency and flatus incontinence.
- Check from delivery records if the woman sustained a third-degree tear.
- Ascertain history of bowel problems:
  - Pre-existing bowel condition, e.g. irritable bowel syndrome, ulcerative colitis
  - Bowel problems associated with pregnancy or previous delivery.

### General advice – All women with bowel problems

- Advise that it is common not to have a bowel motion for 24–48 hours after delivery.
- It is important to stress an adequate intake of fluid and dietary fibre, so that the need for laxatives will be less likely. Laxatives may produce mild abdominal cramps.
- If discomfort from perineal trauma is experienced, adequate analgesia should be taken prior to opening bowels. Paracetamol is the drug of choice: analgesia containing codeine may exacerbate constipation.
- If anxious about passing a bowel motion for the first time after delivery, reassure that this is highly unlikely to result in further perineal damage. It may feel more comfortable if a clean sanitary towel is held against the perineum when passing a motion.

## Management of specific problems

### Constipation

- Establish duration of constipation, whether this occurred in pregnancy, and if it was a common problem prior to pregnancy.
- Check medication the woman is taking for side-effects of constipation. If iron supplementation is being taken, check the most recent Hb result.
- Give general advice as described above, with emphasis on dietary fibre and fluids.
- If these measures do not resolve the constipation and the woman is uncomfortable, a prescription for lactulose should be obtained (non-urgent action). Glycerine suppositories should be used as the next line of management if the woman still has not opened her bowels within 4–5 days of taking lactulose. This should be discussed with the woman, and if she agrees with this treatment, administer the suppositories in accordance with prescription regulations. Review the following day. If the woman feels that the constipation has still not resolved, discuss this and refer (non-urgent action).
- Constipation is associated with anal fissure so be alert for this, particularly if the woman reports severe pain or blood loss on defaecation.

### Haemorrhoids

- It is appropriate to assess the perianal area to confirm a diagnosis of haemorrhoids since other symptoms, in particular anal fissure or blood loss following the passing of a hard stool, could be misdiagnosed as 'haemorrhoids'.
- Ask about onset (ante- or postnatal) and severity. Explain that haemorrhoids are common, and that conservative treatment is usually appropriate. Women should be advised that haemorrhoids may bleed following a bowel movement, but bleeding is generally *painless* unless very severe. A woman who experiences *painful* bleeding may have an anal fissure, and this should be checked.
- If on examination the haemorrhoid is purple, severe, swollen and cannot be manually returned to the anal canal, the woman should be referred (urgent action). A woman may have a less acute, thrombosed haemorrhoid which may not require immediate referral, but if this does not resolve within 2 weeks, referral should be made (non-urgent action).
- All women should be advised to avoid/treat constipation by dietary means and by obtaining a prescription for lactulose if dietary measures do not resolve constipation.
- If painful, topical applications of haemorrhoid creams (i.e. Anusol) may provide some pain relief.
- If the woman reports persistent bleeding after initial treatment for haemorrhoids, she should be referred for clinical assessment (urgent action).

### Faecal incontinence

- If the woman has loss of bowel control, determine if this is flatus, urgency (not being able to defer a bowel movement), soiling or staining of underwear or frank incontinence. If frank incontinence of liquid or solid stool, refer (urgent action).
- Ask about symptoms of constipation (if constipation is severe, incontinence may be due to overflow). If overflow is suspected, referral should be made for advice about treatment owing to the potential severity of constipation (urgent action).
- If the woman reports soiling, initially advise on perianal hygiene following a bowel movement, particularly if she has haemorrhoids. If soiling is not associated with this, refer (urgent action).
- Review regularly – if symptoms do not resolve within about two weeks of onset, after discussion with the woman, referral should be made (non-urgent action). Women with severe incontinence may require referral to a colorectal surgeon for possible secondary repair.
- Women who have a third degree tear should have their perineum examined at regular intervals to ensure that the wound is healing.
- Check that the woman is taking adequate pain relief, which should be paracetamol. If this is not easing pain, refer for stronger analgesia (non-urgent action).
- Ask if lactulose was prescribed for the woman when she was discharged home. If it was, advise on the importance of adhering to the prescription to avoid constipation. If not, refer for a prescription (non-urgent action). Ideally the woman should take the lactulose for two weeks.
- Advice on dietary intake of fibre and fluids should also be stressed especially if stronger analgesia has been prescribed. If constipation is severe and/or the woman is uncomfortable, referral should be made (urgent action).
- Stress the importance of perianal hygiene and if there are concerns about infection of the tear, referral should be made (urgent action).

## SUMMARY GUIDELINE

# Bowel problems

### Initial assessment

- Ask if/when bowels opened since delivery
- Identify specific difficulties (constipation, haemorrhoids, faecal incontinence)
- Check if there is third-degree tear
- Ascertain relevant history, e.g. pre-existing bowel conditions

**Urgent action is required if:**

- Severe constipation
- Persistent bleeding from haemorrhoid
- Severe, swollen haemorrhoid (fourth degree)
- Frank faecal incontinence
- Soiling
- Infection

## What to do

### Constipation

- Advise dietary intake of fibre and fluids and give other general advice
- If not resolved, try lactulose
- If still not resolved, try glycerine suppositories
- If still not resolved and uncomfortable, refer (non-urgent action)

### Haemorrhoids

- Recommend Anusol to all
- Assess whether: fourth degree (remain outside anal canal) – immediate referral (urgent action); third degree (prolapsed but can be manually replaced) – if advice taken and not resolved in 2 weeks, refer (non-urgent action); first/ second degree (less severe) – if advice taken, remains unresolved and is uncomfortable, refer (non-urgent action)

### Faecal incontinence

- Frank incontinence: refer immediately (urgent action)
- Urgency/flatus: if not resolved within 2 weeks, refer (non-urgent action)

### Soiling/Staining

Ascertain presence of haemorrhoids and/or anal fissure. If 'Yes', treat as appropriate. If 'No', advise re constipation and perianal hygiene. If not resolved within 2 weeks, refer (non-urgent action)

## Third-Degree tear

- Check lactulose and antibiotics have been prescribed
- Stress importance of perianal hygiene
- Assess perineal healing and severity of pain
- If no healing progress within 2 weeks or pain persistent, refer (non-urgent action)

## General advice

- It is common not to have a bowel motion for a few days after delivery
- Advise on high-fibre diet and adequate fluid intake
- If there is perineal pain, recommend analgesia (no codeine) before attempting to pass a motion

# References

Abramowitz L, Sobhani I, Ganansia R et al 2000 Are sphincter defects the cause of incontinence after vaginal delivery? Results of a prospective study. Dis Colon Rectum 43: 590-596

Al-Mufti R, McCarthy A, Fisk N 1997 Survey of obstetricians' personal preference and discretionary practice. Eur J Obstet Gynecol Reprod Biol 73: 1-4

Alonso-Coello P, Guyatt G, Heels-Ansdell D et al 2006 Laxatives for the treatment of haemorrhoids. Cochrane Database of Systematic Reviews, Issue 4. Update Software, Oxford

Andrews V, Sultan AH, Thakar R et al 2006 Risk factors for obstetric anal sphincter injury: a prospective study. Birth 33: 117-122

Ansara D, Cohen M, Gallop R et al 2005 Predictors of women's physical and health problems after childbirth. J Psychosom Obstet Gynecol 26: 115-125

Assassa L, Dallosso S, Perry C et al and the Leicestershire MRC Incontinence Study Team 2000 The association between obstetric factors and incontinence: a community survey. Br J Obstet Gynaecol 107: 822

Brown S, Lumley J 1998 Maternal health after childbirth: results of an Australian population based survey. Br J Obstet Gynaecol 105: 156-161

Chaliha C, Sultan AH, Bland J et al 2001 Anal function: effect of pregnancy and delivery. Am J Obstet Gynecol 185: 427-432

Chiarelli P, Murphy B, Cockburn J 2003 Fecal incontinence after high-risk delivery. Obstet Gynecol 102: 1299-1305

Cook T, Mortensen N 1998 Management of faecal incontinence following obstetric injury. Br J Surg 85: 293-299

Donnelly V, Fynes M, Campbell D et al 1998 Obstetric events leading to anal sphincter damage. Obstet Gynecol 92(6): 955-961

Faltin D, Boulvain M, Floris L et al 2005 Diagnosis of anal sphincter tears to prevent fecal incontinence. Obstet Gynecol 106: 6-13

Fernando R, Sultan AH, Kettle C et al 2006 Methods of repair for obstetric anal sphincter injury. Cochrane Database of Systematic Reviews, Issue 3

Fitzpatrick M, Behan M, O'Connell P et al 2003 Randomised clinical trial to assess anal sphincter function following forceps or vacuum assisted vaginal delivery. Br J Obstet Gynaecol 110: 424-429

Fynes M, Donnelley V, O'Connell P et al 1998 Cesarean delivery and anal sphincter injury. Obstet Gynecol 92(4): 496-500.

Fynes M, Marshall K, Cassidy M et al 1999 A prospective, randomized study comparing the effect of augmented biofeedback with sensory biofeedback alone on fecal incontinence after obstetric trauma. Dis Colon Rectum 42(6): 753-761

Garcia J, Marchant S 1993 Back to normal? Postpartum health and illness. In: Thomson A, Robinson S, Tickner V (eds) Research and the Midwife Conference Proceedings 1992. University of Manchester

Glazener C, Abdalla M, Stroud P et al 1995 Postnatal maternal morbidity: extent, causes, prevention and treatment. Br J Obstet Gynaecol 102: 282-287

Glazener C, Herbison G, Wilson P et al 2001 Conservative management of persistent postnatal urinary and faecal incontinence: randomised controlled trial. BMJ 323: 593-596

Glazener CMA, Herbison GP, MacArthur C et al 2005 Randomised controlled trial of conservative management of postnatal urinary and faecal incontinence: six year follow up. BMJ 330: 337-339

Groutz A, Fait J, Lessing M et al 1999 Incidence and obstetric risk factors of postpartum anal incontinence. Scand J Gastroenterol 34: 315-318

Hibbard B 1988 Principles of obstetrics. Butterworths, London

Jewell D, Young G 2001 Interventions for treatment of constipation in pregnancy. Cochrane Database of Systematic Reviews, Issue 2.

Kamm M 1998 Faecal incontinence. BMJ 316: 528-532

MacArthur C, Lewis M, Knox E 1991 *Health after childbirth*. HMSO, London

MacArthur C, Bick D, Keighley M 1997 Faecal incontinence after childbirth. Br J Obstet Gynaecol 104: 46-50

MacArthur C, Glazener C, Wilson P et al 2001 Obstetric practice and faecal incontinence three months after delivery. Br J Obstet Gynaecol 108: 678-683

MacArthur C, Glazener C, Wilson P et al 2005 Faecal incontinence and mode of first and subsequent delivery: a six year longitudinal study. Br J Obstet Gynaecol 112: 1075-1082

MacRae H, McLeod R 1995 Comparison of haemorrhoidal treatment modalities: a meta-analysis. Dis Colon Rectum 38(7): 687-694

Mahony R, Malone P, Nalty J et al 2004 Randomized clinical trial of intra-anal electromyographic biofeedback augmented with electrical stimulation of the anal sphincter in the early treatment of postpartum fecal incontinence. Am J Obstet Gynecol 191: 885-890

Mazouni C, Bretelle F, Battar S et al 2005 Frequency of persistent anal symptoms after first instrumental delivery. Dis Colon Rectum 48: 1432-1436

National Institute for Health and Clinical Excellence (NICE) 2006 Postnatal Care: NICE Clinical Guideline 37. Routine postnatal care of women and their babies.

Nelson R, Westercamp M, Furner S 2006 A systematic review of the efficacy of cesarean section in the preservation of anal continence. Dis Colon Rectum 49: 1587-1595

Oberwalder M, Connor J, Wexner S 2003 Meta-analysis to determine the incidence of obstetric anal sphincter damage. Br J Surg 90: 1333-1337

Peschers U, Sultan AH, Jundt K et al 2003 Urinary and anal incontinence after vacuum delivery. Eur J Obstet Gynecol 110: 39-42

Pfenninger J 1997 Modern treatments for internal haemorrhoids. BMJ 314: 1211-1212

Pollack J, Nordenstam J, Brismar S et al 2004 Anal incontinence after vaginal delivery: a five-year prospective cohort study. Obstet Gynecol 104: 1397-1402

Quijano C, Abalos E 2005 Conservative management of symptomatic and/or complicated haemorrhoids in pregnancy and the puerperium. Cochrane Database of Systematic Reviews, Issue 3

Sartore A, Pregazzi R, Bortoli P et al 2003 Effects of epidural analgesia during labor on pelvic floor function after vaginal delivery. Acta Obstet Gynecol Scand 82: 143-146

Saurel-Cubizolles M-J, Romito P, Lelong N et al 2000 Women's health after childbirth: a longitudinal study in France and Italy. Br J Obstet Gynaecol 107: 1202-1209

Schytt E, Lindmark G, Waldenstrom U 2004 Symptoms of stress incontinence 1 year after childbirth: prevalence and predictors in a national Swedish sample. Acta Obstet Gynecol Scand 83: 928-936

Shelton M 1980 Standardised senna in the management of constipation in the puerperium - A clinical trial. South Afr Med J; 57: 78-80

Shepherd J 2004 Confirming pregnancy and care of the pregnant woman. In: Henderson C, Macdonald S (eds) Mayes' midwifery. Baillière Tindall, London

Signorello L, Harlow B, Chekos A et al 2000 Midline episiotomy and anal incontinence: retrospective cohort study. BMJ 320: 86-90

Sleep J, Grant A 1987 Pelvic floor exercises in postnatal care. Midwifery 3: 158-164

Sultan AH, Stanton S 1996 Preserving the pelvic floor and perineum during childbirth – elective caesarean section? Br J Obstet Gynaecol 103: 731-734

Sultan AH, Kamm M, Hudson C et al 1993 Anal-sphincter disruption during vaginal delivery. N Engl J Med 329(26): 1905-1911

Sultan AH, Kamm M, Hudson C et al 1994 Third degree obstetric anal sphincter tears: risk factors and outcome of primary repair. BMJ 308: 887-891

Sultan AH, Kamm M, Hudson C 1995 Obstetric perineal trauma: an audit of training. J Obstet Gynaecol 15: 19-23

Swash M 1993 Faecal incontinence – childbirth is responsible for most cases. BMJ 307: 636

Thompson J, Roberts C, Currie M et al 2002 Prevalence and persistence of health problems after childbirth: associations with parity and method of birth. Birth 29: 83-94

Tramonte S, Brand M, Mulrow C et al 1997 The treatment of chronic constipation in adults: a systematic review. J Gen Intern Med 12(1): 15-24

van Brummen H, Bruinse H, van de Pol G et al 2006 Defacatory symptoms during and after the first pregnancy: prevalences and associated factors. Int Urogynecol J 17: 224-230

Walsh C, Mooney E, Upton G et al 1996 Incidence of third-degree perineal tears in labour and outcome after primary repair. Br J Surg 83(2): 218-221

Wilson P, Herbison R, Herbison G 1996 Obstetric practice and the prevalence of urinary incontinence three months after delivery. Br J Obstet Gynaecol 103: 154-161

Wood J, Amos L, Rieger N 1998 Third degree anal sphincter tears: risk factors and outcome. Aust NZ J Obstet Gynaecol 38(3): 414-417

Yao G, Albon E, Adi Y et al 2006 A systematic review and economic model of the clinical and cost-effectiveness of immunosuppressive therapy for renal transplantation in children. Health Technol Assess 10: 49

Zetterström J, López A, Anzén B et al 1999 Anal incontinence after vaginal delivery: a prospective study in primiparous women. Br J Obstet Gynaecol 106: 324-330

Chapter **7**

# Depression and other psychological morbidity

## INTRODUCTION

Psychological disturbances following childbirth vary in their timing of onset, duration and severity. Three main conditions are generally described: 'the blues', depression and puerperal psychosis (Kendall-Tackett & Kantor 1993). This guideline deals mainly with depression as the most common manifestation of postpartum psychological morbidity of clinical significance. Although postnatal blues are more widely experienced, this is a transient condition and generally of minor importance. Puerperal psychosis is rare but is serious and requires urgent referral for treatment, so must be recognised by the midwife. Other less common psychological conditions which may be experienced by postpartum women, such as stress reactions, anxiety disorders, and disorders of the mother–infant relationship, will not be referred to in this guideline.

There is increased concern that much psychiatric morbidity around the time of childbirth remains unidentified. The last three UK *Reports on confidential enquiries in maternal deaths* – now called *Saving mother's lives: Reviewing maternal deaths to make motherhood safer* (Lewis 2007) – have included a chapter on deaths from psychiatric causes. Suicide and death from other psychiatric causes was the most common cause of indirect maternal death and the largest cause overall.

# POSTNATAL DEPRESSION

## Definition

Postnatal depression (PND), although sometimes difficult to define and recognise, was described in the classic study by Pitt in 1968 as: 'what lies
between the extreme of severe puerperal depression, with the risk of suicide
and infanticide, and the trivial weepiness of "the blues"; something occurring frequently, much less dramatic than the former, yet decidedly more dis-
abling than the latter' (p. 1325). There is no precise definition of postnatal
depression, but its clinical features are similar to depression occurring at
any time within the general population and include lethargy, tearfulness,
oversensitivity, hopelessness, anxiety, guilt, irrational fears and disturbed
sleep patterns. The typical gradual onset means that it may not be easily dis-
tinguishable from the fatigue and emotional lability experienced by most
mothers as they recover from childbirth and adjust to the demands of the
baby (Holden 1991).

The *International classification of diseases* (ICD) (WHO 1990) makes provision for a diagnosis of puerperal mental health disorder if occurring postpartum and cannot be otherwise classified, and the *Diagnostic and
Statistical Manual of Mental Disorders* (DSM-IV) (American Psychiatric Association Task Force 2000) allows postpartum onset to be specified for mood disorders that have started within 4 weeks postpartum. However, in both
clinical practice and research, a much wider time frame is used to define
postnatal depression, often including onset in the antenatal period and for
up to a year postpartum. The Scottish Intercollegiate Guidelines Network
(SIGN) defines postnatal depression as any non-psychotic depressive illness of mild to moderate severity occurring during the first postnatal year
(SIGN 2002).

## Frequency of occurrence

There have been at least two well-conducted systematic reviews and metaanalyses of the prevalence of depression in the postpartum period. O'Hara
& Swain (1996), in a meta-analysis of 59 studies that included assessment
using either standardised psychiatric interview-based methods or validated
self-report measures, found the estimated average prevalence of postpartum
depression to be 12.8%. They found that prevalence estimates were affected
by the length of the postpartum period under evaluation and by the nature
of the assessment method. In general, the self-report measures produced
higher estimates; for example, average prevalence in 12 studies using the
Edinburgh Postnatal Depression Scale (EPDS) was 12%, 11.6% in eight using
the Beck Depression Inventory (BDI) and 18% in five using the Center for
Epidemiological Studies-Depression Scale (CES-D). Average prevalence
based on the interview-based methods was, for example, 10.5% in 19 studies
using the Research Diagnostic Criteria (RDC) and 7.2% in three studies using
the DSM.

A more recent meta-analysis of 28 prospective studies, based only on structured clinical interview assessments, estimated point prevalence including both major and minor depression at various times during the first postpartum year to be between 6.5% and 12.9% (Gavin et al 2005). In 18 of the studies prevalence was assessed by conducting a clinical interview on all study women, and in 10 studies women first completed a self-report instrument, with a clinical interview in those scoring above the predetermined cut-off. This review calculated point prevalence and period prevalence. Point prevalence of major and minor depression was found to rise after delivery and to be highest in the third month postpartum, at 12.9%. In the fourth to seventh months, prevalence declined slightly, staying in the range 9.9–10.6%, after which it declined to 6.5%. Each of these estimates, however, is based only on a few studies so all have wide confidence intervals. There were fewer estimates for period prevalence, the best estimate being that as many as 19.2% of women may have major or minor depression in the first 3 months after delivery, but confidence intervals were wide.

Although the term 'postnatal depression' is commonly used by professionals and mothers, some researchers have questioned the extent to which it comprises a specific entity (Green 1998). The review by Gavin et al (2005) identified three prevalence studies that had comparison groups of similar aged non-childbearing women (Cooper et al 1988, Cox et al 1993, O'Hara et al 1990). None of these indicated a statistically significant difference for prevalence of major or minor depression. Only one of these studies (Cox et al 1993) examined incidence of depression and this showed a threefold higher rate of depression within the first 5 weeks of childbirth amongst the postnatal women, compared with the equivalent time period for control women (odds ratio (OR) 3.26, 95% confidence interval (CI) 1.17–9.06). At 6 months postpartum, however, the difference in incidence was less and was not statistically significant (OR 1.48, 95% CI 0.77–2.82). Cox et al (1993) concluded that the threefold excess within the first month is most likely as a result of the 'life event' of giving birth and the immediate impact of a new family member, and that the category of PND remains a useful diagnostic term. Whether or not the prevalence, duration and nature of depression after childbirth are similar to those occurring among women generally, its appearance after birth remains relevant to those involved in providing maternity services.

## Risk factors

In the search for possible risk factors of PND, studies have examined a large number of maternal, obstetric and sociodemographic characteristics, in particular, obstetric interventions, sociodemographic characteristics, psychiatric history, interpersonal relationships and support, and hormone disorders. There have been three systematic reviews of the risk factors of PND. O'Hara & Swain (1996) found that the strongest predictors of postpartum depression were past history of psychopathology and psychological disturbance during pregnancy, poor marital relationship and low social support and stressful life events. They found that indicators of low social status showed a small but significant predictive relationship with depression and there was a weak association with obstetric complications. Beck (2001) updated a previous meta-analysis of predictors of postpartum depression, first published in 1996 (Beck 1996), as there had been many more studies. She identified 13 significant predictors of depression, with 10 regarded as strongly predictive. These were prenatal depression, low self-esteem, childcare stress, prenatal anxiety, depression history, life stress, social support, poor marital relationship, difficult infant temperament and maternity blues. Marital status, low socio-economic status and unplanned/unwanted pregnancy were moderate predictors. Robertson et al (2004) completed the most recent systematic review, and gave risk factors in order of magnitude of effect size. These were depression or anxiety during pregnancy, life events, poor social support, previous history of depression, neuroticism and poor marital relationship. Low socio-economic status and obstetric factors had small effect sizes.

The NICE (2007) guidelines on antenatal and postnatal mental health, in a review of risk factors, comment on the lack of overlap of the studies that were included in the three reviews. The guidelines also consider a weakness of the reviews to be the inclusion of studies with PND based on only self-report scales in addition to diagnostic interviews. The review by Beck (2001) has more of the former than the review by O'Hara & Swain (1996). Robertson et al (2004) do not define method of assessing depression in their review, other than it had to have 'proven reliability'. The NICE mental health guidelines found eight additional studies published since the reviews, thus not included in them, and comment that these largely support the findings of the earlier studies.

There is no good evidence that hormonal changes are a risk factor for PND (Romito 1990, SIGN 2002). A recent review specifically examining the possible link between caesarean section and postpartum depression concluded that such a link has not been established (Carter et al 2006).

## Additional effects

Postnatal depression has been shown to have consequences for the development of the child, with some effects demonstrable in the longer term. Prospective studies have found an association between PND and insecure infant attachment (Murray 1992), behavioural and emotional problems in early childhood (Caplan et al 1989), cognitive development (Coghill et al 1986, Hay et al 2001, Sharp et al 1995) and later psychiatric and behavioural outcomes (Halligan et al 2007, Hay et al 2003). Cooper & Murray (1998), in a review of PND, proposed that the association between PND and adverse child development was as a consequence of an impaired pattern of communication between the woman and her infant. That PND might have a lasting impact on a woman and her infant highlights the importance of the early detection and management of this problem.

An Australian study of 1336 women followed up at 6–7 months postpartum (Brown & Lumley 2000) found a positive association between PND (EPDS 13 or more) and maternal physical health and postpartum recovery. Similar associations were shown in a more in-depth telephone interview of a subsample of women at 7–9 months.

## Management

The management of PND will depend on its severity, but can consist of pharmacological or various forms of psychological or supportive treatments or a combination of these. For a very small proportion of women, admission to a specialised unit will be necessary. Since the last edition of this book there have been several systematic reviews of effects of treatment of PND (Boath & Henshaw 2001, Dennis 2004, Hoffbrand et al 2001, Lumley et al 2004), and in the UK there have been guidelines produced by SIGN in 2002 and by NICE in 2007. In view of this, the individual management trials will not be described and the focus will be on the most recent systematic reviews and guidelines.

### Non-pharmacological therapies

In the systematic review by Lumley et al (2004) these were categorised into 'universal' (provided to the whole group), 'selective' (provided to high-risk women) and 'indicated' (provided to those identified as depressed or probably depressed). Since this chapter is about treatment of PND rather than prevention, the latter category is relevant here. The conclusions of this review, based on 11 randomised controlled trials of 'indicated' postnatal interventions, were that there is strong evidence that postnatal counselling interventions, provided to women with depression or probable depression, by professionals from a variety of backgrounds after specific training, will reduce depressive symptoms and depression substantially. The types of interventions in the various trials included non-directive counselling, cognitive behaviour therapy (CBT), interpersonal psychotherapy (IPT), psychodynamic therapy, psychosocial/educational support and physical therapy (massage, relaxation).

Dennis (2004) categorised interventions in her systematic review of non-biological interventions (which also included non-randomised treatment studies) according to type of intervention. She concludes in relation to CBT that, due to methodological limitations, there is limited evidence regarding the inclusion of this approach in the treatment of postpartum depression, although the results of these studies are primarily beneficial. For interpersonal psychotherapy, the results from one well-designed trial and smaller studies support the recommendation that IPT may be effective in the treatment of PND. She notes that conclusions about the relative effectiveness of most of the non-biological treatments cannot be reached, since most trials were compared with standard care.

The NICE guidelines on antenatal and postnatal mental health (2007) categorise studies into comparisons of non-pharmacological interventions with standard care/wait list control and comparisons of one type of intervention with another. In relation to the former, based on eight RCTs, they conclude that there is an effect on depression symptoms of targeted treatments, particularly in trials with a formal diagnosis of depression. Treatments with at least moderate-quality evidence that show a positive effect include CBT, IPT, psychodynamic therapy and non-directive counselling. For differential effectiveness of the various non-pharmacological treatments only four trials were found, and the NICE conclusions are that evidence on this is limited. Physical non-pharmacological treatments are reviewed separately, which include exercise, acupuncture and infant massage, with one very small study for each. Since exercise, however, has also been examined in non-postnatal populations, they conclude that this is worth considering in managing women with mild to moderate PND.

## Pharmacological therapy

The NICE guidelines (2007) found three RCTs examining antidepressant therapy for PND, one comparing this with placebo and counselling (Appleby et al 1997) and the others each comparing two different antidepressant drugs (Misri et al 2004, Wisner et al 2006). The guidelines conclude that there is some evidence of the efficacy of antidepressants, particularly of fluoxetine (with a single session of counselling), although fluoxetine with six sessions of counselling was only as effective as the counselling sessions alone, and some evidence from uncontrolled studies. There was no evidence of superior efficacy of sertraline over nortryptyline. They conclude that both the number of trials and included participants are low but the findings are consistent with those from non-postnatal populations.

Oestrogen therapy for the treatment of postpartum depression was examined in one small RCT, and NICE (2007) concluded that this showed some evidence in favour of treatment compared with placebo. A Cochrane systematic review of oestrogens and progestins for preventing and treating postpartum depression was more cautious on its conclusions about this: oestrogen therapy may be of modest value for the treatment of severe postpartum depression (Dennis et al 1999).

## Methods of identifying postnatal depression

There has been much discussion since the first edition of this book about whether and how health professionals should systematically identify or screen for PND. The Edinburgh Postnatal Depression Scale (EPDS) (Cox et al 1987) was developed as a screening instrument specifically for postpartum women and was increasingly used in the 1990s, mainly by health visitors. The EPDS is a 10-item scale, each item having four possible responses, and the woman is asked to choose the response that comes closest to how she has felt during the previous 7 days. The responses are then scored. A score of 12 or more is considered to identify those women more likely to have depression (Cox et al 1987). The questionnaire had been found to be acceptable to both women and health professionals and to be quick to complete (Holden 1991).

In 2002, however, the National Screening Committee undertook a review of screening for PND and recommended that this should not be undertaken, and that the EPDS should not be used as a screening tool but only alongside clinical judgement. This was mainly because among the six EPDS validation studies some showed the positive predictive value (those correctly identified as having depression from the total with a positive test score) to be relatively low.

The NICE postnatal care guideline, launched in July 2006, and the NICE antenatal and postnatal mental health guideline, launched in February 2007, both address the issue of the identification of PND but have different recommendations for implementation. The postnatal care guideline states 'At each postnatal contact, women should be asked about their emotional well-being, what family and social support they have and their usual coping strategies for dealing with day-to-day matters' (NICE 2006, p. 6). The antenatal and postnatal mental health guideline states that:

> At a woman's first contact with primary care, at her booking visit and postnatally (usually at 4–6 weeks and 3–4 months), healthcare professionals (including midwives, obstetricians, health visitors and GPs) should ask two questions to identify possible depression:
>
> - During the past month, have you often been bothered by feeling down, depressed or hopeless?
> - During the past month, have you often been bothered by having little interest or pleasure in doing things?
>
> A third question should be considered if the woman answers 'yes':
>
> - Is this something you feel you need or want help with? (NICE 2007, p. 13).

These questions were devised by Whooley et al (1997) and tested in a general population sample. The guideline later suggests that 'health care professionals may consider the use of self-report measures such as the EPDS, HADS or PHQ-9 as part of a subsequent assessment or for the routine monitoring of outcomes'.

The reason why the NICE antenatal and postnatal mental health guidelines do not recommend use of the EPDS as a screening tool is because the positive predictive value of the test varies considerably across studies, from 33% to 93%. The Whooley et al (1997) questions, however, have a similarly low positive predictive value, at 32%, and have never been tested in an antenatal or postnatal population. Indeed, the guideline proposes that a priority area for research is a validation study of these questions against a psychiatric interview in women in the first postpartum year. It would therefore seem premature to recommend them as standard care and this has resulted in concern that their use may discourage the detection of postpartum depression (Coyne & Mitchell 2007).

Given that this is all very recent, it is difficult to know exactly what should be recommended in terms of how PND should be identified, although it is clear that health professionals should do this systematically in one way or another. In summary, therefore, health professionals in their consultations with postpartum women should check whether the woman seems to be depressed in whatever way is considered to be appropriate, probably based on local practice and always including clinical judgement.

## POSTPARTUM BLUES

The transient and frequent experience of weepiness and mood instability is known as the postpartum blues (Romito 1990). It is a syndrome experienced a few days after the delivery, typically between about the third and tenth days. The exact definition of 'the blues' varies to some extent (Kennerley & Gath 1989, O'Hara et al 1991) but the most commonly reported symptoms include tearfulness, lability of mood, irritability and sometimes headache (Snaith 1983, O'Hara et al 1991, Hannah et al 1992, Piper 1992). Observational studies have found the prevalence of the blues to range from 50% to 80% (Kendall et al 1981, Stein et al 1981, George & Sandler 1988, Henshaw et al 2004). They are considered to be self-limiting and no specific treatment is required, although reassurance is sometimes needed. Some studies have found an association between the blues and PND (O'Hara et al 1991, Beck et al 1992, Henshaw et al 2004), although a plausible hormonal basis to account for this link has not been identified (O'Hara et al 1991, Murray 1992).

## PUERPERAL PSYCHOSIS

The most severe form of postnatal psychiatric morbidity is puerperal psychosis and this is also the most uncommon. It is characterised by thought disorders and/or severe depression and may even result in suicide or infanticide. The midwife's role is particularly important in the early recognition of severe psychiatric disturbance, as these symptoms must be managed quickly and appropriately.

The prevalence of psychotic illness in the puerperium is about 1 in 500 births (Kendall et al 1987). A recent review of the literature on postpartum psychosis notes that the onset occurs in the first 1–4 weeks after birth (Sit et al 2006). Protheroe (1969) found that 94% of puerperal psychosis had an onset within 4 weeks of childbirth, 65% within 2 weeks. A sudden onset, after an interval of well-being since the birth, is characteristic (Riley 1995, Thurtle 1995). Women who have had previous puerperal psychosis have a risk of between 25% and 57% of a future puerperal episode and the risk of a non-puerperal episode is even higher (SIGN 2002).

Puerperal psychosis may be characterised by schizophrenic and affective symptoms (Riley 1995). Sit et al (2006) note that the woman typically develops frank psychosis, cognitive impairment and grossly disorganised behaviour that represents a complete change from previous functioning. Hospitalisation is usually necessary and it is preferable to admit the woman and her infant together to a specialist unit. There is limited evidence on the management of specifically puerperal psychosis, but the SIGN guideline (2002) notes that, since it is essentially an affective psychosis, treatments used for this within general populations are appropriate. These include antidepressant, mood-stabilising or neuroleptic drugs, and electroconvulsive therapy (ECT) may occasionally be used (Riley 1995, SIGN 2002). Further research is required of the most appropriate management of childbirth-related psychosis.

## POSTNATAL DEBRIEFING

In the late 1990s there was much discussion in midwifery journals and text-books about whether there is a need to 'debrief' women of their labour and delivery experiences in order to prevent psychological morbidity (Ralph & Alexander 1994, Abbott et al 1997), although there was limited evidence on this (Alexander 1998, 1999). Debriefing generally involves the promotion of a form of emotional 'catharsis' by encouraging recollection of the traumatic event. It is often offered as an intervention following serious incidents to prevent posttraumatic stress disorder (PTSD), although a Cochrane review has shown no evidence from non-postpartum populations of benefit from a single debriefing session (Rose et al 2002). There have now been seven RCTs that have investigated debriefing-type interventions in postnatal populations and effects on subsequent depression. A further RCT investigated effects on fear of childbirth but not depression (Kershaw et al 2005). Most of the RCTs have found no evidence of any effect of 'debriefing' on subsequent depression.

Some trials recruited selected samples of 'high-risk' postpartum women. An Australian study by Small et al (2000) recruited 1041 women who had caesarean section, forceps or vacuum extraction deliveries, randomised to an intervention of an hour of debriefing during the postnatal hospital stay by a trained midwife or standard care. Initial follow-up was at 6 months postpartum (Small et al 2000), and just over half the sample were followed again at 4–6 years (Small et al 2006), at neither time showing any difference in EPDS-assessed depression. Ryding et al (2004) recruited 162 women who had an emergency caesarean section delivery who were randomised to two sessions of group counselling or routine care control and found no difference between groups in EPDS-assessed depression at 6 months. Tam et al (2003) recruited 560 women who had 'unexpected antenatal, intrapartum or post-partum events leading to suboptimal outcomes' who were randomised to one-to-one educational counselling or standard care. There were no differences at 6 weeks or 6 months postpartum in depression assessed by the Hospital Anxiety and Depression Scale (HADS). Gamble et al (2005) recruited women prior to birth and then screened them within 72 hours of birth for PTSD and recruited those positive for this, which was just under one-third of the initial sample. Among the 50 women randomised to counselling (provided at 72 hours and 4–6 weeks postpartum), 16 women had an EPDS score indicating probable depression, compared with 18 of the 53 women in the standard care group, whilst by 3 months postpartum the respective numbers with a high score were four compared with 17 women, a statistically significant difference.

A study by Priest et al (2003) recruited 1745 women who had delivered a healthy term infant who were randomised to a single session of critical incident stress debriefing with 72 hours of birth or standard care. Follow-up at 2, 6 and 12 months postpartum showed no differences in depression assessed by EPDS at any follow-up period. A smaller trial by Selkirk et al (2006) included 149 women randomised to a 30–60 minute session of debriefing by a specially trained midwife within 3 days postpartum or standard care. There were no differences in EPDS scores between groups at 1 or 3 month follow-up. Lavender & Walkinshaw (1998) included 120 women randomised to a 30–120 minute debriefing session given by a midwife on the postnatal ward after day 2 or routine care. Follow-up was at 3 weeks postpartum using the HADS, at which time the intervention group had significantly lower anxiety and depression scores. The HADS has not been validated for use on postpartum women and a commentary on the study suggested that the debriefing and short follow-up may have been measuring women's experience of the 'blues' rather than depression (Wessely 1998).

In summary, the evidence on postnatal debriefing indicates that this will have no benefit to women in terms of reducing PND, and neither the NICE postnatal care (NICE 2006) nor the NICE antenatal and postnatal mental health (NICE 2007) guidelines recommend that it be undertaken.

## SUMMARY OF THE EVIDENCE USED IN THIS GUIDELINE

- Systematic reviews including numerous studies have shown depression to occur in the postpartum period in 7–13% of women, depending on methods of assessment used.
- Adverse effects of maternal depression on the child are well documented.
- The main risk factors for PND are previous psychopathology, in pregnancy or at other times, poor marital or partner relationship, low social support and stressful life events. Hormonal changes and caesarean section do not impose increased risk. There is a lack of consensus for other possible risk factors.
- There is lack of consensus on how health professionals should identify PND but agreement that some sort of systematic method should be used alongside clinical judgement.
- Evidence from numerous small randomised controlled trials consistently shows that various forms of psychological intervention are effective in treating PND, but larger trials are still required.

- There is little evidence on the effectiveness of antidepressant drug treatment specifically in postnatal women, with its use based on general population evidence. There may be modest benefit of oestrogen in the management of severe PND.
- Evidence from RCTs indicates that there is no evidence to support postnatal debriefing or other forms of counselling in preventing PND.

## WHAT TO DO

### Initial assessment

The main role of the healthcare professional in relation to postpartum psychiatric morbidity is to be alert to its detection using whatever method is locally appropriate.

In addition to being alert to the detection of psychological conditions, it is necessary to be able to distinguish the various manifestations. Table 7.1 summarises the main features of the blues, depression and psychosis.

If at any time the healthcare professional suspects the existence of any other psychological morbidity, such as severe anxiety disorders or stress reactions, the woman should be referred for further evaluation (urgent action).

Table 7.1

|  | Postpartum blues | Postnatal depression | Puerperal psychosis |
|---|---|---|---|
| Frequency | 50–80% | 7–13% | 1 in 500 |
| Symptoms | Tearfulness; irritability; lability of mood; sometimes headache. | Lethargy; tearfulness; oversensitivity; hopelessness; anxiety; guilt; irrational fears; disturbed sleep patterns. | Thought disorders; delusion; confusion; agitation; fear; insomnia; severe depression. Rarely suicide/ infanticide. |
| Onset | Few days after delivery. | Mainly within first month or two of delivery. | Most commonly in first 4 weeks after delivery. |
| Duration | A few days or less. | Most resolve within about 3 months or less, especially with treatment, but can persist. | Variable. |
| Action | Transient condition. No action except reassurance needed unless does not resolve. | If suspected refer (urgent action). | Immediate referral (emergency action). Do not leave woman alone. Explain to family. |

### Woman showing symptoms of depression

- Where there is concern that a woman may be suffering from PND, following discussion with the woman, referral is required (urgent action), and the health visitor should be informed. Relevant members of the healthcare team should liaise closely to plan care.
- Encourage the woman to utilise support of partner (and/or close relative or friend) in helping care for the baby and in talking about her feelings.
- Ensure that the woman knows how to contact the healthcare professional whenever she needs to.
- Conflicting advice should be avoided.
- Offer literature on self-help and details of local and/or national support groups.

### Woman showing symptoms of puerperal psychosis (or if the midwife considers that there is a risk of suicide or child abuse)

- Emergency action required.
- Do not leave the woman alone.
- Explain the situation to the woman and partner.

## SUMMARY GUIDELINE

## Depression and other psychological morbidity

### Initial assessment

- Ask how the woman is feeling
- Be especially aware if:
  - there is a history of psychiatric illness
  - her relationship with her partner is difficult or she is unsupported
  - what appeared to be the blues does not resolve

## What to do

### Woman showing symptoms of depression

- If concerned that a woman may be depressed, discuss and refer (urgent action).
- Encourage support of partner (and/or close relative or friend) in caring for baby.

- Ensure that the woman knows how to contact the midwife and/or health visitor at any time.
- Avoid conflicting advice.
- Offer self-help and support group literature.
- If at any time the healthcare professional suspects the existence of any other psychological morbidity, such as severe anxiety disorders or stress reactions, the woman should be referred (urgent action)

The summary below sets out the main features of the blues, depression and psychosis, and action to be taken by the healthcare professional.

# References

Abbott H, Bick DE, MacArthur C 1997 Health after birth. In: Henderson C, Jones K (eds) Essential midwifery. Mosby, London

Alexander J 1998 Confusing debriefing and defusing postnatally: the need for clarity of terms, purpose and value. Midwifery 14(2): 122-124

Alexander J 1999 Can midwives reduce postpartum psychological morbidity? A randomised controlled trial. MIDIRS Comments. MIDIRS Midwifery Digest 9(3): 370-371

American Psychiatric Association Task Force on DSM-IV 2000 Diagnosis and Statistical Manual of Mental Disorders, 4th edn. American Psychiatric Association, Washington DC

Appleby L, Warner R, Whitton A et al 1997 A controlled study of fluoxetine and cognitive-behavioural counselling in the treatment of postnatal depression. BMJ 314: 932

Beck CT 1996 A meta-analysis of predictors of postpartum depression. Nurs Res 45: 297-303

Beck CT 2001 Predictors of postpartum depression: an update. Nurs Res 50: 275-285

Beck CT, Reynolds M, Rutowski P 1992 Maternity blues and postpartum depression. J Obstet Gynecol Neonatal Nurs 21(4): 287-293

Boath E, Henshaw C 2001 The treatment of postnatal depression: a comprehensive literature review. J Reprod Infant Psychol 19: 215-248

Brown S, Lumley J 2000 Physical health problems after childbirth and maternal depression at six to seven months postpartum. Br J Obstet Gynaecol 107: 1194-1201

Caplan H, Coghill S, Alexandra H et al 1989 Maternal depression and the emotional development of the child. Br J Psychiatry 154: 818-822

Carter F, Frampton C, Mulder R 2006 Cesarean section and postpartum depression: a review of the evidence examining the link. Psychosomatic Med 68: 321-330

Coghill S, Caplan H, Alexandra H et al 1986 Impact of maternal postnatal depression on cognitive development of young children. BMJ 292: 1165-1167

Cooper P, Murrary L 1998 Postnatal depression. Clinical review. BMJ 316: 1884-1886

Cooper P, Campbell E, Day A et al 1988 Non psychotic psychiatric disorder after childbirth. A prospective study of prevalence, incidence, course and nature. Br J Psychiatry 152: 799-806

Cox J, Holden J, Sagovsky R 1987 Detection of postnatal depression. Development of the 10-item Edinburgh Postnatal Depression Scale. Br J Psychiatry 150: 782-786

Cox J, Murray D, Chapman G 1993 A controlled study of the onset, duration and prevalence of postnatal depression. Br J Psychiatry 163: 27-31

Coyne J, Mitchell A 2007 Do NICE recommendations discourage detection of depression in pregnancy and postpartum women? BMJ 5 March 2007. Rapid response to: Mayor S. Guidance recommends asking pregnant women about mental health. BMJ 2007; 334: 445-446

Dennis C-L 2004 Treatment of postpartum depression, Part 2: a critical review of nonbiological interventions. J Clin Psychiatry 65: 1252-1265

Dennis C-L, Ross L, Herxheimer A 1999 Oestrogens and progestins for preventing and treating postpartum depression. Cochrane Database of Systematic Reviews, Issue 3

Gamble J, Creedy D, Moyle W et al 2005 Effectiveness of a counselling intervention after a traumatic childbirth: a randomized controlled trial. Birth 32: 11-19

Gavin N, Gaynes B, Lohr K et al 2005 Perinatal depression. A systematic review of prevalence and incidence. Obstet Gynecol 106; 1071-1083

George A, Sandler M 1988 Endocrine and biochemical studies in puerperal mental disorders. In: Kumar R, Brockington I (eds) Motherhood and mental illness, vol 2. Wright (Butterworths), Cambridge

Green J 1998 Postnatal depression or perinatal dysphoria? Findings from a longitudinal community-based study using the Edinburgh Postnatal Depression Scale. J Reprod Infant Psychol 16(2/3): 143-155

Halligan S, Murray L, Martins C et al 2007 Maternal depression and psychiatric outcomes in adolescent offspring: a 13-year longitudinal study. J Affect Dis 97: 145-154

Hannah P, Adams D Lee A et al 1992 Links between early post-partum mood and post-natal depression. Br J Psychiatry 160: 777-780

Hay D, Pawlby S, Sharp D et al 2001 Intellectual problems shown by 11-year-old children whose mothers had postnatal depression. J Child Psychol Psychiatry 42: 871-889

Hay D, Pawlby S, Angold A et al 2003 Pathways to violence in the children of mothers who were depressed postpartum. Dev Psychology 39: 1083-1094

Henshaw C, Foreman D, Cox J 2004 Postnatal blues: a risk factor for postnatal depression. J Psychosom Obstet Gynecol 25: 267-272

Hoffbrand S, Howard L, Crawley H 2002 Antidepressant treatment for post-natal depression. Cochrane Database of Systematic Reviews, Issue 2

Holden J 1991 Postnatal depression: its nature, effects and identification using the Edinburgh Postnatal Depression Scale. Birth 18(4): 211-221

Kendall R, McGuire R, Connor Y et al 1981 Mood changes in the first three weeks after childbirth. J Affect Disord 3: 317-326

Kendall R, Chalmers J, Platz C 1987 Epidemiology of puerperal psychosis. Br J Psychiatry 150: 662-673

Kendall-Tackett K, Kantor G 1993 Postpartum depression. A comprehensive approach for nurses. Sage, London

Kennerley H, Gath D 1989 Maternity blues: I. detection and measurement by questionnaire. Br J Psychiatry 155: 356-362

Kershaw K, Jolly J, Bhabra K et al 2005 Randomised controlled trial of community debriefing following operative delivery. Br J Obstet Gynaecol 112: 1504-1509

Lavender T, Walkinshaw S 1998 Can midwives reduce postpartum psychological morbidity? A randomised controlled trial. Birth 25: 215-219

Lewis G, Drife J (eds) 2004. Why mothers die 2000–2002. Sixth report of the confidential enquiries into maternal and child health. RCGP Press, London

Lewis G (Ed) 2007 Saving Mothers Lives: Reviewing maternal deaths to make motherhood safer 2003-2005 CEMACH, London

Lumley J, Austin M-P, Mitchell C 2004 Intervening to reduce depression after birth: a systematic review of the randomized trials. Int J Technol Assess Health Care 20: 128-144

Misri S, Reebye P, Corral M et al 2004 The use of paroxetine and cognitive-behaviour therapy in postpartum depression and anxiety: a randomized controlled trial. J Clin Psychiatry 65: 1236-1241

Murray L 1992 The impact of postnatal depression on child development. J Child Psychol Psychiatry 33: 543-561

National Institute for Health and Clinical Excellence (NICE) 2006 Postnatal care: routine postnatal care of women and their babies. Nice Clinical Guideline 37

National Institute for Health and Clinical Excellence (NICE) 2007 Antenatal and postnatal mental health: clinical management and service guidance. NICE Clinical Guideline 45

O'Hara M, Swain A 1996 Rates and risk of postpartum depression – a meta-analysis. Int Rev Psychiatry 8: 37-54

O'Hara M, Zekoski E, Phillipps L et al 1990 Controlled prospective study of postpartum mood disorders: comparison of childbearing and nonchildbearing women. J Abnormal Psychol 99: 3-15

O'Hara MW, Schlechte J, Lewis D et al 1991 Prospective study of postpartum blues. Arch Gen Psychiatry 48: 801-806

Pitt B 1968 'Atypical' depression following childbirth. Br J Psychiatry 114: 1325-1335

Piper M 1992 Emotional and mental disturbances of the puerperium. Midwives Chron Nurs Notes August: 228-235

Priest S, Henderson J, Evans S et al 2003 Stress debriefing after childbirth: a randomised controlled trial. Med J Aust 178: 542-545

Protheroe C 1969 Puerperal psychoses: a long term study. Br J Psychiatry 115(518): 9-30

Ralph K, Alexander J 1994 Borne under stress. MIDIRS Midwif Digest 4(3): 330-332

Riley D 1995 Perinatal mental health: a source book for health professionals. Radcliffe Medical Press, Oxford

Robertson E, Grace S, Wallington T et al 2004 Antenatal risk factors for postpartum depression: a synthesis of recent literature. Gen Hosp Psychiatry 26: 289-295

Romito P 1990 Postpartum depression and the experience of motherhood. Acta Obstet Gynecol Scand 69(suppl): 154

Rose S, Bisson J, Churchill R et al 2002 Psychological debriefing for preventing post traumatic stress disorder (PTSD). Cochrane Database of Systematic Reviews, Issue 2

Ryding E, Wirén E, Johansson G et al 2004 Group counselling for mothers after emergency cesarean section: a randomized controlled trial of intervention. Birth 31: 247-253

Scottish Intercollegiate Guidelines Network (SIGN) 2002 Postnatal depression and puerperal psychosis. A national clinical guideline. Scottish Intercollegiate Guidelines Network, Edinburgh

Selkirk R, McLaren S, Ollerenshaw A et al 2006 The longitudinal effects of midwife-led postnatal debriefing on the psychological health of mothers. J Reprod Infant Psychol 24: 133-147

Sharp D, Hay D, Pawlby S et al 1995 The impact of postnatal depression on boy's intellectual development. J Child Psychol Psychiatry 36: 1315-1337

Sit D, Rothschild A, Wisner K 2006 A review of postpartum psychosis. J Women's Health 15: 352-368

Small R, Lumley J, Donohue L et al 2000 Randomised controlled trial of midwife led debriefing to reduce maternal depression after operative childbirth. BMJ 321: 1043-1047

Small R, Lumley J, Toomey L 2006 Midwife-led debriefing after operative birth: four to six year follow-up of a randomised trial. BMC Med 4: 3

Snaith R 1983 Pregnancy related psychiatric disorder. Br J Hosp Med 29: 450-456

Stein G, Marsh A, Morton J 1981 Mental symptoms, weight change and electrolyte excretion during the first postpartum week. J Psychosom Res 25: 395-408

Tam W, Lee D, Chiu H et al 2003 A randomised controlled trial of educational counselling on the management of women who have suffered suboptimal outcomes in pregnancy. Br J Obstet Gynaecol 110: 853-859

Thurtle V 1995 Post-natal depression: the relevance of sociological approaches. J Adv Nurs 22: 416-424

Wessely S 1998 Commentary: reducing distress after normal childbirth. Birth 24(4): 220-221

Whooley M, Avins A, Miranda J et al 1997 Case-finding instruments for depression. Two questionnaires are as good as many. J Gen Internal Med 12: 439-445

Wisner K, Hanusa B, Perel J 2006 Postpartum depression. A randomised trial of sertraline versus nortriptyline. J Clin Psychopharmacol 26: 353-360

World Health Organization (WHO) 1990 International Classification of Diseases, 10th revision. World Health Organization, Geneva

# Chapter 8

# Fatigue

## INTRODUCTION

Fatigue is a non specific symptom shown in general population studies to be experienced at some time by many people. Women in these studies commonly report higher rates of fatigue than men (Chen 1986, Cox et al 1987). It is a well-recognised problem anecdotally after childbirth, and although few studies have specifically investigated this, widespread and persistent symptoms have been reported (Bick & MacArthur 1995, MacArthur et al 1991). These studies found that fatigue was underreported to health professionals, as women expect to experience it when caring for a new baby and consider it to be a normal reaction to the physiological changes of childbirth. However, it is likely that the duration and severity of postnatal fatigue will determine whether for some women it has a significant effect on their health (Rubin 1975). There has been increasing interest in issues related to the definition and diagnosis of chronic fatigue syndrome (CFS), which is also more likely to be experienced by women (Department of Health 2002). However, the main focus of this chapter is postnatal fatigue as a reaction to recently giving birth (referred to as 'simple fatigue' in the 'What to Do' section).

## Definition

The simplest definition of fatigue is probably that of the physiologist – a decrease in response after prolonged activity. Fatigue is a protective mechanism whereby the body slows down or stops so that overuse is prevented and regeneration can take place. No direct correlation has been described between the level of fatigue experienced and energy expenditure or stress.

Individual coping style, physical fitness, psychological make-up and motivation may mean that one person will feel fatigued when others do not (Hart et al 1990). Fatigue is primarily a subjective experience which incorporates psychological and environmental factors and is to be expected in certain situations: after excessive physical exertion or following prolonged wakefulness without adequate sleep. One definition of fatigue used widely in nursing research is that of the North American Nursing Diagnosis Association (NANDA): 'An overwhelming sustained sense of exhaustion and decreased capacity for physical and mental work' (NANDA 1990; see also Lee et al 1994, Milligan & Pugh 1994, Piper 1989).

The difficulty in classification of fatigue as abnormal or excessive is compounded following childbirth, when care of an infant inevitably results in increased activity and disturbed sleep patterns, and care should be taken when eliciting the range and onset of symptoms in a woman who has recently given birth.

## Frequency of occurrence

Various instruments measuring subjective fatigue have been developed – Symptom Distress Scale, Yoshitake's Fatigue Scale, Rhoten Fatigue Scale, Pearson Byars Fatigue Feeling Tone Scale – but none has gained widespread acceptance as a standard objective measure of fatigue (Hart et al 1990). There have also been recent developments in validated self-rating scales developed to assess symptoms of CFS, including the CDC Symptom Inventory (Wagner et al 2005). The most common method of documenting prevalence of fatigue in studies of postpartum women continues to be a tick box response to a question asking whether the woman has experienced fatigue or extreme tiredness, usually within a list of symptoms.

The wording of this question will influence the morbidity identified. The question may be worded to establish whether the symptom is new, with scope to record previous experience of the symptom, onset in relation to the birth, duration and whether medical help had been sought and received (MacArthur et al 1991). Asking women about health symptoms which have been a problem will elicit positive responses only from those who do not assume some degree of the problem to be normal after childbirth (Brown & Lumley 1998). Questions worded to establish point prevalence without attempting to determine if this is a new symptom will include those in whom it predates childbirth and exclude those who did have the symptom which has now resolved (Saurel-Cubizolles et al 2000). Importance is sometimes assessed in postpartum studies by relating rates of fatigue to those for other health symptoms after childbirth, but attribution of cause and effect in cross-sectional data is impossible (Gardner & Campbell 1991).

High rates of fatigue are to be expected, and have been reported in the early postpartum period. Early studies, of small numbers of women, described high rates of concern about fatigue among women at 4 and 6 weeks postpartum (Fawcett & York 1986). Tulman & Fawcett (1988) found that, of 70 women who had delivered a full-term infant within the previous 5 years, only 51% reported that they had regained their usual level of energy by 6 weeks postpartum. The authors suggested that the traditional view of recovery from childbirth being complete at 6 weeks postpartum needed to be reconsidered. This was a small study in which the sampling method limits generalisability: the majority of women were recruited at a conference for members of a caesarean section prevention movement. In another small qualitative study, Ruchala & Halstead (1994) also found that at 2 weeks after discharge from hospital, 76% of 50 postpartum women interviewed cited fatigue as a major physical concern. Fatigue was an underlying theme for the women, and being tired was a major descriptor of their postpartum experiences for 44%.

The first broad-based sample to describe persistence of fatigue and other health problems well beyond 6 weeks was by MacArthur et al (1991). In a West Midlands study of over 11,000 women, questioned 1–9 years after they had given birth, 17.1% of women reported extreme tiredness, as they perceived it, occurring within 3 months of delivery and lasting for more than 6 weeks. In 12.2% of the sample, the women had not experienced tiredness this extreme before. For 6.1% of the sample, the fatigue had persisted for more than a year. The association between childbirth and persistent fatigue was confirmed in a further, more detailed study, which necessitated shorter recall (Bick & MacArthur 1995). Of 1278 women surveyed at 6–7 months after delivery, 41% reported extreme tiredness occurring for the first time within 3 months of the delivery and lasting for over 6 weeks. The majority of these women reported the symptoms of fatigue as persistent.

Similar findings were described by Glazener et al (1995), in a prospective observational study of a 20% sample (n = 1249) of women who delivered in 1 year in the Grampian region of Scotland. Women were surveyed about health problems at discharge from hospital, at 8 weeks and, for half of the sample, again at 12–18 months postpartum. Tiredness was reported by 42% of women at discharge, 59% up to 8 weeks and 54% between 2 and 18 months postpartum. In an Australian study of health among 1336 women delivered in 1993 and surveyed at 6–7 months postpartum, 69.4% reported tiredness/exhaustion occurring as a problem some time since the birth (Brown & Lumley 1998). A postal questionnaire survey for the Audit Commission (Garcia et al 1998), of a sample of 2406 women throughout England and Wales at 4 months postpartum, asked about health problems as part of a wider study of maternity care. The women were asked to think back to 10 days, 1 month and 3 months and say which of a number of health problems they had at those times: 43% reported having had fatigue at 10 days, 31% at 1 month and 21% at 3 months. None of these studies attempted to establish whether the symptoms reported were new in the postpartum period.

Recall of between 6 weeks and 9 years was required in these studies but the findings are consistent with those from more recent prospective studies estimating point prevalence of various health problems at 5 and 12 months

(Saurel-Cubizolles et al 2000) and at 12 months only (MacArthur et al 2003), although prevalence rates differ. In the longitudinal survey of the health of 697 Italian and 589 French women delivered in 1993–94, tiredness was reported by 46.1% Italian and 48.4% French women at 5 months postpartum (Saurel-Cubizolles et al 2000). By 12 months these figures had increased to 60.7% and 67.5% respectively. In a large cluster randomised controlled trial (RCT) of a new model of midwifery-led postnatal care, women were asked about the presence of a number of health symptoms at 12 months after giving birth (MacArthur et al 2003). Overall, of 1512 women, 414 (27%) reported fatigue.

These assessments have been able only to determine the presence or absence of fatigue with some attempt to delineate its duration. In a Canadian study Smith-Hanrahan & Deblois (1995) used the Rhoten Fatigue Scale (a visual analogue scale ranging from not tired to totally exhausted) to measure present fatigue intensity in subjects reporting fatigue at 2–3 days, 1 week and 6 weeks postpartum. The aim of the study was to examine the effect of early discharge on maternal fatigue and ability to perform activities of daily living, but difficulties experienced in enacting the randomisation mean that comparisons between arms in this study are unlikely to be sound. For the study population as a whole, however, some level of fatigue was recorded on the Rhoten Scale in 95% of the 81 mothers at the time of discharge from hospital. At 6 weeks postpartum, this figure was 86%. Sufficient detail is not given in the paper to determine the overall proportion with severe tiredness at each assessment point but it appears to be around 20% of all women.

Self-reported fatigue is entirely subjective but as described earlier, a standard objective measure is not available. In a study designed to examine the extent, severity and effect of postnatal symptoms, fatigue was commonly reported (Bick & MacArthur 1995). Of 1278 women who completed a postal questionnaire, 523 (40%) reported fatigue and of these, 77% (n = 405) reported that it impacted on their lives in some way. Women reported that fatigue affected their ability to concentrate, they felt bad-tempered or did not want to socialise. Interestingly, it did not appear to affect their ability to care for their infant. Postnatal fatigue was associated with problems related to resuming sexual intercourse in the eight week and at 12–18 month follow-up of women who participated in the study of postnatal health in the Grampian region of Scotland (Glazener 1997). In a prospective cohort study from Sweden which investigated the prevalence of physical symptoms among 2413 women at 2 months and 1 year after birth, women's reporting of their health as 'low' was associated with symptoms affecting physical functioning and well-being, including self-reports of fatigue (Schytt et al 2005).

All these surveys will be subject to some degree of response bias. In addition, such studies have limited ability to place the person's reported level of fatigue within their physical, psychological, work and social context. In studies where more detailed evidence of fatigue was sought, or where a more multidimensional view of fatigue was explored, the small size and non-random sampling methods used limit their generalisability (Gardner 1991).

Finding an appropriate comparison group to determine if fatigue prevalence is higher in postpartum women than in other groups is complex. Gjerdingen & Froberg (1991) compared adoptive mothers (6 weeks after adoption) and biological mothers (7 weeks after delivery) with a non-pregnant control group who had attended for pelvic examination. Both adoptive and biological mothers reported more fatigue than controls but the generalisability and validity of the comparison are very limited. Of 444 women with a mean age of 38, attending a general practice in London, 12% were suffering from 'chronic fatigue' (Anthony et al 1990). Of the 167 men in the study (mean age 41) the figure was 9%. Sampling methods and the predominantly middle-class composition of the sample limit generalisability of these findings. In a Norwegian population-based random sample of 3500 people, 11.4% of all women (aged 19–80 years) reported substantial fatigue lasting 6 months or longer (Loge et al 1998). In a US survey of a national probability-based sample of adults aged 25–74 years (the size of the sample and response rates are not quoted), 20.4% of women reported suffering from fatigue, compared to 14.3% of men.

## Risk factors

Pugh & Milligan (1993) categorised potential factors in predisposing a woman to childbearing fatigue as physical, psychological and situational. Physical factors may be normal physiological changes or pathological ones, which in the postpartum period can include effects of mode of delivery, anaemia, infection and haemorrhage (Chen 1986, Paterson et al 1994). Psychological factors might include the mother's reaction to childbearing and mental states such as anxiety and depression. Situational factors may be personal, such as parity, age, method of feeding and sleep patterns, or environmental, including socio-economic status, social support and lifestyle.

### Physical risk factors

Delivery factors identified in the study by MacArthur et al (1991) as independent risk factors for long-term fatigue included multiple pregnancy, longer first stage of labour, inhalation anaesthesia and postpartum haemorrhage but not operative delivery. Milligan et al (1990) did show a significant association between caesarean section and fatigue in a group of 259 women surveyed before discharge from hospital, but when the same women were surveyed at 6 weeks and 3 months, no significant effect was seen. Findings from the other two large studies previously quoted are consistent with an early excess for caesarean section which diminishes over time. At 12–18 months fatigue was not associated with caesarean section in Glazener's study, but there was an association in the reports of fatigue at 0–13 days and at up to 8 weeks (Glazener 1995). Tiredness was more common in women delivered by caesarean section and surveyed at 6–7 months in Brown & Lumley's study (1998) but the effect was not statistically significant (Brown & Lumley 1998). The other studies have not reported on the other delivery factors.

Few studies have examined the physiological determinants of postnatal fatigue, but Paterson et al (1994) investigated the impact of a low (<10.5 g/dl) haemoglobin (Hb) on the postnatal mental and physical health of 1010 women. Hb results were obtained at 'booking', 34 weeks, third day post-delivery and at 6 weeks postpartum. Women were asked to complete questionnaires about their health at 10 days, 4 weeks and 6 weeks after delivery on their health. Full data including Hb were obtained from only 52% of the original sample. A low Hb on day 3 was more likely to be diagnosed in younger women (aged under 25); among primiparae; women who had had operative or instrumental delivery; women who had a low Hb at 34 weeks gestation; and those with a blood loss of over 250 ml recorded at delivery. Some of these variables are interrelated (for example, parity and mode of delivery) but statistical analysis to determine independence of effect was not undertaken. Women with a low Hb at day 3 were significantly more likely to report feeling low in energy in the questionnaire at day 10. They also were more likely to report being breathless; faint and dizzy; to have painful sutures and tingling of the fingers or toes. By 6 weeks no difference was apparent between groups with and without low Hb, but it is not clear from the paper what action was taken on the basis of the Hb result, though it is apparent that some of the women in the study were taking iron supplements.

Other physical problems worth considering if a woman reports extreme tiredness are infections and, though much less common, thyroid disorders and cardiomyopathy (Atkinson & Baxley 1994). CFS, a syndrome where persistent fatigue is felt and significant disability experienced without apparent cause, may affect women after childbirth, but no studies have reported rates of occurrence in this group. There is ongoing debate about the most appropriate diagnostic criteria for CFS, with two commonly cited definitions, the Oxford criteria and the US Centers for Disease Control and Prevention criteria, both stating that debilitating fatigue must be present for at least 6 months, that there is some functional impairment and that this is not associated with any other identifiable condition (Fukuda et al 1994, Sharpe et al 1991). These definitions do differ, however, in the number and severity of symptoms which must be present. In a general population study of fatigue, Chen (1986) found heavier women more likely to be fatigued than lighter ones (based on body mass index).

## Psychological risk factors

Fatigue is a well-recognised symptom of depression though it may be difficult to clarify whether anxiety and depression are the cause or result of fatigue (Unterman et al 1990). Of 1065 postpartum women who reported depression in MacArthur et al's 1991 study, 47% (496) also reported extreme tiredness. These 496 women constituted 35% of all women (1427) who reported extreme tiredness. In Brown & Lumley's (2000) survey of 1336 Australian women at 6–7 months postpartum, tiredness was 3.4 times more likely to be reported by women with scores on the Edinburgh Postnatal Depression Score indicating probable depression. Ansara and colleagues (2005) undertook a study in Toronto to examine the extent and correlates of common physical health symptoms in women 2 months after giving birth. Women were recruited from six Toronto area hospitals and interviewed by telephone 8–10 weeks later. Of 332 women approached, 200 (60%) were interviewed. Most women (96%) reported at least one physical health problem at 2 months. Stepwise logistic regression analysis showed that a self-reported history of antenatal depression was a significant predictor of excessive fatigue after giving birth.

Gardner (1991) collected data by questionnaire at 2 days, 2 weeks and 6 weeks postpartum from 35 of 68 randomly selected American women. The sample were only mildly fatigued, as scored on the Rhoten Fatigue Scale, and fatigue and depression scores were significantly, but not strongly, correlated at 2 days and 2 weeks, but not at 6 weeks postpartum. Milligan et al (1990) found that comparatively little of the variation in fatigue at 6 weeks and 3 months postpartum was explained by other factors in models which controlled for depression.

The correlation between fatigue symptoms and psychiatric disorder has also been demonstrated in general population studies of patients with CFS. In a nested case–control study, 60% of 214 chronic fatigue patients were found to have a current psychiatric disorder compared to 19% of 214 matched controls (Wessely et al 1996).

It is difficult to determine causal association between fatigue and depression, although evidence from prospective studies indicates that sleep disruption may be a risk factor for postnatal depression. Dennis & Ross (2005) examined relationships between infant sleep patterns, maternal fatigue and the development of postnatal depression in women with no major depressive symptomatology at 1 week after giving birth; 505 women who had an EPDS score of <13 at 1 week after giving birth completed a questionnaire at 4 and 8 weeks. Those women who had EPDS scores of >12 at 4 and 8 weeks were significantly more likely to report that their babies cried often, that they were woken three times or more between 10pm and 6am, received less than 6 hours of sleep in a 24-hour period over the previous week, and considered their baby's sleep pattern did not allow them to get a reasonable amount of sleep. The researchers concluded that infant sleep patterns and maternal fatigue were associated with the onset of depression after birth, and preventive interventions should be designed to reduce sleep deprivation in the first few weeks after birth. It is also possible that women experiencing depression may be more likely to overreport crying and waking in their babies.

## Situational risk factors

There have been contrasting findings with regard to a possible association between fatigue and parity. MacArthur et al (1991) found fatigue more common in older primiparae. Glazener et al (1995) and Brown & Lumley (1998) found no association with parity and did not report on an effect of age. In Gardner's small study (n = 35), older women reported less fatigue but the sample selection, response rate and overall low levels of fatigue in this study diminish its generalisability and power.

The method of infant feeding may have an impact on postnatal fatigue. Two studies found breastfeeding more likely to be associated with fatigue than bottlefeeding (MacArthur et al 1991, Milligan & Pugh 1994). In a small non-random convenience sample, breastfeeding problem severity was associated with fatigue in each assessment at 3 days, 3, 6 and 9 weeks postpartum (Wambach 1998). A recent qualitative study highlighted that the desire of healthcare professionals to protect women from tiredness or distress may result in them recommending supplementation of infants with artificial or expressed breast milk, which may result in early cessation of breastfeeding (Cloherty et al 2004). Data were collected from 30 mothers and 17 midwives, and a smaller number of neonatal nurses (n = 4), members of the medical staff (n = 6) and healthcare assistants (n = 3). Mothers who planned to breastfeed, but were supplementing their babies, were invited to take part. One of the themes generated related to conflict in the midwives' role to support breastfeeding with their desire to protect women from tiredness or distress, a theme confirmed by the mothers' accounts. In some cases, the midwives suggested supplementation and in some cases, it was requested by the mother. The importance of midwives being aware of other solutions to assist tired and distressed breastfeeding mothers should be a priority.

With the trend in earlier discharge from hospital, a few small studies have attempted to explore the effect on women's health. In their qualitative study, Ruchala & Halstead (1994) linked comments that several women made about hospital stay being too short with the importance of fatigue underlying many issues. Smith-Hanrahan & Deblois (1995) attempted to randomise 125 women into early and 'traditional' discharge groups and to compare fatigue levels at three intervals in the first 6 weeks postpartum. Implementation was impractical as 29 of 67 women randomised to receive traditional care were discharged early due to bed shortages. The study, subject to other methodological weaknesses, was analysed in three groups, but no differences in fatigue levels were demonstrated. Using a rest and activity questionnaire, Carty et al (1996) failed to show a difference in fatigue at 1 and 4 weeks postpartum, between women discharged in 3 days or sooner with those who stayed in hospital longer.

Oakley (1992) proposed that changes in the social circumstances of women during the last decade, such as increasing numbers of lone-parent families, lack of support, and the need to continue in paid employment, were likely to lead to fatigue in the new mother. MacArthur et al (1991) showed higher reports of extreme tiredness in unmarried women. In the European survey women were asked to describe their relationship with their partner. At 12 months postpartum, rates of extreme tiredness in lone mothers in both countries were lower than all cohabiting groups except those who described their relationship as very good (Saurel-Cubizolles et al 2000). It has been suggested that diversity of social support can act as a buffer to the stress of maternal fatigue on parenting (Parks et al 1992).

Classification of socio-economic status in postpartum women is difficult and little evidence of an effect on postpartum fatigue has been shown. Among the 35 women in Gardner's study (1991), fatigue at 6 weeks postpartum was negatively correlated with the mother's education level but, as mentioned earlier, the generalisability of these results is limited for reasons discussed above. In Saurel-Cubizolles' study (2000) tiredness at 12 months postpartum was reported more frequently by women with a severe financial problem, though only for French women was the difference statistically significant (70.5 vs 60.9; $p<0.02$). Tiredness was reported more often for women employed at 12 months postpartum in this study, though again the effect was statistically significant only for French women (70.5% vs 60.9%).

## Management

Fatigue is common postpartum, but it is also a major feature of many illnesses. It is important that any medical conditions associated with fatigue should be identified and treated. In Paterson et al's (1994) study of postpartum anaemia, as well as symptoms of fatigue at 10 days, women with a low Hb at day 3 were more likely to report being breathless; faint and dizzy; to have painful sutures and tingling of the fingers or toes. Slightly more women with a low Hb at day 3 scored 14 or more on the EPDS at day 10 (10% vs 7%), although this was not statistically significant. It does suggest that symptom assessment and EPDS results may be of use in discriminating physiological causes of fatigue. Anaemia in postpartum women may remain undetected, as many obstetric units do not perform routine postnatal Hb. Predictors of low postpartum Hb in Paterson's study have already been quoted and could help in diagnosing anaemia as a cause of postpartum fatigue.

Given the association between fatigue and anxiety and depression, it is important to exclude psychological illness in fatigued patients.

In the absence of a physical or psychological cause for postpartum fatigue, it is widely assumed that nothing can be done. No studies of effectiveness of management strategies for postpartum fatigue were identified. The NICE postnatal care guideline recommendations for persistent fatigue include that women should be offered advice on diet, exercise and planning activities (NICE 2006); however, these recommendations were based on evidence from general population studies. Management strategies for fatigue in general population groups can be broadly divided into those where sufferers are advised to limit the demands placed on their bodies and those geared around a graded increase in activity. The strategy of limiting demand amounts to treating fatigue as a protective symptom against overstressing the body. In trying to increase activity, the association between inactivity and increased levels of fatigue is assumed to be causal (Chen 1986). Some literature exists in relation to the management of CFS but since a major component of this disorder is significant disability with no apparent cause, applicability to postpartum women is limited (Fulcher & White 1997, Price & Couper 2000).

It is possible that the level of postnatal care a woman received after birth will impact on her levels of fatigue. In the cluster RCT undertaken by MacArthur and colleagues (2003), women who had received the new model of midwifery-led postnatal care were significantly less likely to report fatigue at 12 months (OR 0.75, 95% CI 0.60–0.94). Symptoms of interest had been included on checklists used by the intervention midwives at 10 and 28 days and 3 months postpartum to assist the identification of common health problems, with accompanying guidelines to enable the midwife to implement appropriate management. That the main trial outcomes showed a difference in psychological health based on the mental health component score of the SF36 and the EPDS, but no difference in physical health, may indicate that the difference in fatigue (a secondary outcome) was mediated through benefit to psychological health. Even with no difference in physical health outcomes, it is still possible that early acknowledgement of these and appropriate support from the midwife could have had a positive impact on levels of fatigue.

Strategies suggested for the management of fatigue targeted at individuals are not specific to postpartum women, and draw on data, often qualitative, from studies of fatigued patients with serious medical illnesses such as cancer or on no data at all (Hart et al 1990, Piper 1989). Nonetheless, in the absence of good evidence of effective management, some of the recommendations from these papers are included.

Given the potential association between fatigue and psychological factors, therapeutic listening, counselling and patient education to reduce anxiety and increase their sense of control are proposed (Piper 1989).

Hart et al (1990) suggest that management should be based on the individual being able to influence her own health, and that she should have an active role in decisions about treatment. By increasing the woman's awareness of the possible problems of the puerperium, she can be advised on changing behaviour to overcome or minimise the effects of fatigue, for example by taking a rest after feeding the infant.

To help the woman recognise sources of excessive energy consumption, it is suggested that they maintain a fatigue diary for 1 week (Hart et al 1990). Recording a detailed diary may not be feasible for postpartum women but it might help them to review their activities with a view to conserving energy. Several short periods of rest are postulated to be more beneficial than one long period (Hart et al 1990). The latter method is more realistic for the postpartum mother, who is likely to be able to find short periods to rest rather than a long period. Symptoms of fatigue may reflect underlying marginal nutritional deficiency (Hart et al 1990), and the importance of a well-balanced diet should be discussed, particularly with lactating mothers. Calorific intake is also important.

Exercise has been associated with improvement in mood, level of tension, anxiety, psychological functioning and depression whilst physical deconditioning may be caused by reduced physical activity which may accentuate physical and psychological effects (Fulcher & White 1997). Achieving an appropriate pattern of activity and rest is problematic for the postpartum woman and energy needs to be conserved. It may be that in the immediate postnatal period, exercise should be limited to maintenance of function and support of daily activities.

Natural techniques for relieving fatigue are also discussed by Hart et al (1990). These include progressive muscle relaxation, acupressure, reflexology, massage, relaxation imagery and visualisation, but evidence is required of their benefit for postnatal women.

## SUMMARY OF THE EVIDENCE USED IN THIS GUIDELINE

- Fatigue is a non-specific symptom assessed subjectively. General population studies show it is common and prevalence rates are high among postpartum women.
- In the absence of a standard objective measure of fatigue, prevalence among postpartum women has usually been ascertained by asking women about extreme tiredness as one of many postnatal health problems.
- Observational studies of self-reported postnatal health problems show that for many women, fatigue can become a chronic symptom and for some, it will affect other aspects of their life.
- It is important to identify and manage any underlying psychological or physical illness that may present with fatigue.
- Advice on how to incorporate adequate rest periods into their daily routine and to ensure they maintain adequate nutritional intake may help women to reduce their fatigue levels.
- Women who are breastfeeding should not be offered supplementary infant formula feeds due to concerns about their level of fatigue, as this may be associated with early cessation of breastfeeding (refer to Chapter 4 for evidence on support for breastfeeding women).
- An RCT of planned, tailored and extended postnatal care showed a beneficial impact on a woman's experience of fatigue at 12 months postpartum.

## WHAT TO DO

### Initial assessment for women with fatigue

- Exclude depression. Symptoms to be aware of are: lethargy; tearfulness; anxiety; guilt; irritability; disturbed sleep patterns; lack of energy; poor appetite; poor concentration. If depression is suspected refer to guideline on Depression and Other Psychological Morbidity (Chapter 7).
- Exclude anaemia. Ask about breathlessness, dizziness, tingling in fingers and toes. Check haemoglobin level. If low, treat as local policy.
- Consider and exclude possibility of infection, thyroid disorder or other physical or medical problems. If any are identified, use appropriate guideline if available or refer as appropriate (urgent action).
- If there are no underlying conditions give general advice as below.

### 'Simple' fatigue

- Help the woman plan her time each day to include short periods of rest. It may be appropriate to suggest that she asks a relative or friend to help with household tasks so that she has more time to spend caring for her baby.
- Explain that exercise may be helpful. For example, a short walk each day at a time when the mother feels she has most energy, such as in the morning, could be followed by a short period of rest.
- Check that dietary intake is adequate and stress the need to eat at regular intervals.
- Where appropriate discuss social circumstances and lifestyle (e.g. young single mother). If the woman feels it necessary, referral to an appropriate healthcare professional may be arranged, if additional social support would be beneficial.
- Encourage the woman to discuss any problems or worries she may have with the midwife and/or a close friend or family member.
- If the woman is breastfeeding suggest that she use the side-lying position for at least some of the feeds.
- It may be helpful if the woman keeps a 'diary' of daily tasks for 1 week to assess if fatigue is related to any particular activity or time of day. Her activities can then be reviewed in relation to this.
- Review symptoms at subsequent visits. If symptoms are severe and/or persist, referral should be made for further assessment (urgent action).
- Referral to the appropriate healthcare professional should be made if concerned about well-being at any time.

## SUMMARY GUIDELINE

# Fatigue

### Initial assessment

- Exclude depression. Symptoms to be aware of are: lethargy; tearfulness; anxiety; guilt; irritability; disturbed sleep patterns; lack of energy; poor appetite; poor concentration. If depression is suspected refer to guideline on Depression and Other Psychological Morbidity (Chapter 7)
- Exclude anaemia. Ask about breathlessness, faintness, dizziness, tingling in fingers and toes. Check haemoglobin level. If low, treat as local policy
- Exclude other physical or medical problems. If any are identified use appropriate guideline if available or refer for assessment (urgent action)

## What to do

### 'Simple' fatigue

- Help the woman plan her time each day to include short periods of rest. If possible ask a relative or friend to help
- Check that dietary intake is adequate and stress need to eat regularly
- Where appropriate discuss social circumstances and lifestyle (e.g. young single mother). Referral should be arranged, if additional social support would be beneficial
- Explain importance of exercise. Advise short daily walk when the woman feels she has most energy, which should then be followed by a short period of rest
- Encourage the woman to discuss any problems or worries she may have with the midwife and/or a close friend or family member
- It may be helpful if the woman keeps a diary of daily tasks to assess if fatigue is related to any particular activity or time of day and help her plan activity to include rest periods
- Review symptoms at subsequent visits. If symptoms are severe and/or persist, refer as appropriate (urgent action)
- Refer if concerned about well-being at any time

## References

Ansara D, Cohen M, Gallop R et al 2005 Predictors of women's physical health problems after childbirth. J Psychosom Obstet Gynecol 26(2): 115-125

Anthony D 1990 Tired, weak, or in need of rest: fatigue among general practice attenders. BMJ 301:1199-1202

Atkinson L, Baxley E 1994 Postpartum fatigue Am Fam Phys 50(1): 113-118

Bick DE, MacArthur C 1995 The extent, severity and effect of health problems after childbirth. Br J Midwif 3(1): 27-31

Brown S, Lumley J 1998 Changing childbirth: lessons from an Australian survey of 1336 women. Br J Obstet Gynaecol 105(2): 143-155

Brown S, Lumley J 2000 Physical health problems after childbirth and maternal depression at six to seven months postpartum. Br J Obstet Gynaecol 107: 1194-1201

Carty E, Bradley C, Winslow W 1996 Women's perceptions of fatigue during pregnancy and postpartum: the impact of length of hospital stay. Clin Nurs Res 5(1): 67-80

Chen M 1986 The epidemiology of self-perceived fatigue among adults. Prevent Med 15: 74-81

Cloherty M, Alexander J, Holloway I 2004 Supplementing breast-fed babies in the UK to protect their mothers from tiredness or distress. Midwifery 20(2): 194-204

Cox B, Blaxter M, Buckle A et al 1987 The health and lifestyles survey. Health Promotion Research Trust, London

Department of Health 2002 A report of the CFS/ME working group: report to the Chief Medical Officer of an Independent Working Group. Department of Health, London

Dennis C, Ross L 2005 Relationships among infant sleep patterns, maternal fatigue and development of depressive symptomatology. Birth 32(3): 187-193

Fawcett J, York 1986 Spouses' physical and psychological symptoms during pregnancy and the portpartum. Nurs Res 45: 144-148

Fukuda K, Straus S, Hickie I et al 1994 The chronic fatigue syndrome: a comprehensive approach to its definition and study. International Chronic Fatigue Syndrome Study Group. Ann Intern Med 12(12): 953-959

Fulcher KY, White PD 1997 Randomised controlled trial of graded exercise in patients with the chronic fatigue syndrome. BMJ 314: 1647-1652

Garcia J, Redshaw M, Fitzsimons B et al 1998 First class delivery. A national survey of women's views of maternity care. Audit Commission Publications, Abingdon, Oxford

Gardner D 1991 Fatigue in postpartum women. Appl Nurs Res 4(2): 57-62

Gardner D, Campbell B 1991 Assessing postpartum fatigue. Am J Matern Child Nurs 16(5): 264-266

Gjerdingen D, Froberg D 1991 Predictors of health in new mothers. Social Sci Med 33(12): 1399-1407

Glazener C 1997 Sexual function after childbirth: women's experiences, persistent morbidity and lack of professional recognition. Br J Obstet Gynaecol 104: 330-335

Glazener C, Abdalla M, Stoud P et al 1995 Postnatal maternal morbidity: extent, causes, prevention and treatment. Br J Obstet Gynaecol 102(4): 282-287

Hart L, Freel M, Milde F 1990 Fatigue. Nurs Clin North Am 25(4): 967-976

Lee K, Lentz M, Taylor D et al 1994 Fatigue as a response to environmental demands in women's lives. IMAGE: J Nurs Sch 26(2): 149-154

Loge J, Ekeberg O, Kassa S 1998 Fatigue in the general Norwegian population: normative data and associations. J Psychomatic Res 45(1): 53-65

MacArthur C, Lewis M, Knox E 1991 Health after childbirth. HMSO, London

MacArthur C, Winter H, Bick DE et al 2003 Redesigning postnatal care; a randomised controlled trial of protocol based, midwifery led care focused on individual women's physical and psychological health needs. NHS R and D, NCC HTA. Vol. 7. No. 37.

Milligan R, Pugh L 1994 Fatigue during the childbearing period. Annu Rev Nurs Res 12: 33-49

Milligan R, Parks P, Lenz E 1990 An analysis of postpartum fatigue over the first three months of the postpartum period. In: Wang J, Simoni PA, Nath C (eds) Vision of excellence: the decade of the nineties. West Virginia Nurses' Association Research Conference Group, Charleston, West Virginia

National Institute for Health and Clinical Excellence (NICE) 2006 Routine postnatal care of women and their babies. Postnatal Care: NICE Clinical Guideline 37

North American Nursing Diagnosis Association (NANDA) 1990 Taxonomy I revisited – 1990, with official nursing diagnoses. CV Mosby, St Louis, Misssouri

Oakley A 1992 The changing social context of pregnancy care. In: Chamberlain G, Zander L (eds) Pregnancy care in the 1990s. Parthenon, Carnforth, Lancs

Parks P, Lenz E, Jenkins L 1992 The role of social support and stressors for mothers and infants. Child Care Health Dev 18(3): 171

Paterson J, Davis J, Gregory M et al 1994 A study of the effects of low haemoglobin on postnatal women. Midwifery 10: 77-86

Piper B 1989 Fatigue: current bases for practice. In: Funk S, Tornquist E, Champagne M et al (eds) Management of pain, fatigue and nausea. Springer, New York

Price J, Couper J 2000 Cognitive behaviour therapy for chronic fatigue syndrome in adults. Cochrane Database of Systematic Reviews, Issue 3

Pugh L, Milligan R 1993 A framework for the study of childbearing fatigue. Adv Nurs Sci 15(4): 60-70

Rubin R 1975 Maternity nursing stops too soon. Am J Nurs 75:1680-1684

Ruchala P, Halstead L 1994 The postpartum experience of low-risk women: a time of adjustment and change. Maternal-Child Nurs J 22(3): 83-89

Saurel-Cubizolles M-J, Romito P, Lelong N et al 2000 Women's health after childbirth: a longitudinal study in France and Italy. Br J Obstet Gynaecol 107: 1201-1209

Schytt E, Lindmark G, Waldenstrom U 2005 Physical symptoms after childbirth: prevalence and association with self-rated health. Br J Obstet Gynaecol 112(2): 210-217

Sharpe M, Archard L, Banatvala J et al 1991 A report – chronic fatigue syndrome: guidelines for research. J Roy Soc Med 84(2): 118-121

Smith-Hanrahan C, Deblois D 1995 Postpartum early discharge: impact on maternal fatigue and functional ability. Clin Nurs Res 4(1): 50-66

Tulman L, Fawcett J 1988 Return of functional ability after childbirth. Nurs Res 37(2): 77-81

Unterman R, Posner N, Williams K 1990 Postpartum depressive disorders: changing trends. Birth 17: 131-137

Wagner D, Nisenbaum R, Heim C et al 2005 Psychometric properties of the CDC Symptom Inventory for assessment of chronic fatigue syndrome. Population Health Metrics 3:8

Wambach K 1998 Maternal fatigue in breastfeeding primiparae during the first nine weeks postpartum. J Hum Lactation 14(3): 219-229

Wessely S, Chalder T, Hirsch S et al 1996 Psychological symptoms, somatic symptoms and psychiatric disorder in chronic fatigue and chronic fatigue syndrome: a prospective study in the primary care setting. Am J Psychiatry 153(8): 1050-1059

Chapter **9**

# Backache

## CHAPTER CONTENTS

## INTRODUCTION

Women commonly experience backache during pregnancy and following delivery. Postpartum studies have not generally specified types of backache, but it is likely that most is simple backache.

## SIMPLE BACKACHE

### Definition

'Simple' backache is the term used to describe back pain which is musculo skeletal in origin, mechanical in nature, varies with physical activity and time and can affect the lumbosacral region, buttocks and thighs in a person who is generally well. The lower back is the most commonly reported site of pain (MacArthur et al 1991, Östgaard & Anderson 1992, Russell et al 1993, Turgut et al 1998).

### Frequency of occurrence

Backache is very common during pregnancy, affecting 50% or more of all women to varying degrees (Berg et al 1988, Fast et al 1987, Östgaard & Anderson 1991) It is thought to be triggered by hormonal factors and the increased weight of the gravid uterus (MacLennan et al 1986). Several studies have also shown backache to be common following childbirth, with a prevalence range of 20–50% varying according to definition and timing. MacArthur et al (1991), in a study of 11,701 postnatal women questioned

1–9 years after the birth, found that 23% reported backache that had started within 3 months of giving birth and lasted for longer than 6 weeks, with 14% reporting this as a new symptom. Many more reported postpartum backache but could not accurately date these symptoms. Brown & Lumley (1998), in an Australian study of health problems among 1336 women at 6–7 months postpartum, found that backache was reported as a problem at some time since the birth by 44% of this sample.

Several longitudinal studies have found that postpartum backache is often not transient. Östgaard & Anderson (1991, 1992), in a Swedish cohort study, followed a representative sample of 817 women through pregnancy, at the end of which 67% reported back pain and at 12–18 month follow-up back pain prevalence was 37%. A 20% sample (n = 1249) of all women who delivered during 1 year in one health region of Scotland were given a questionnaire about health problems in hospital, then a postal questionnaire at 8 weeks postpartum, half receiving another at 12–18 months, to investigate subsequent problems. Backache was reported by 22% of the women in hospital, by 24% between then and 8 weeks, and by 20% after this (Glazener et al 1993). Among 1042 women delivering in a maternity unit in Boston, USA, 44% reported backache at 1–2 months postpartum (Breen et al 1994). At 12–18 month follow-up, rates had not changed, with 49% experiencing back pain during the preceding 3 months (Groves et al 1994). At the time of follow-up, backache was more common (66%) among the women who had reported backache in the 1–2 month questionnaire, compared with those who had not (21%). A longitudinal study of the health of postpartum women in France (n = 589) and Italy (n = 697), followed at 5 and 12 months, found a high prevalence of backache in each country at both times: 49% and 50% in France, and 47% and 65% in Italy. The Italian rates showed a surprising increase over the time (Saurel-Cubizolles et al 2000).

A postal questionnaire survey for the Audit Commission (Garcia et al 1998), of a population-based sample of 2406 women throughout England and Wales at 4 months postpartum, asked about health problems as part of a wider study of maternity care. The women were asked to think back to 10 days, 1 month and 3 months postpartum and say which of a number of health problems they had at those times: 35% reported having had backache at 10 days, 27% at 1 month and 28% at 3 months.

A few studies have examined the severity of postpartum back pain. Bick & MacArthur (1995) investigated the severity and effect of various morbidities, including backache, in a sample of 1278 women by postal questionnaire at 6–7 months postpartum. There were 582 women (46%) who reported backache (new and recurrent) occurring within 3 months of birth and lasting for longer than 6 weeks; 49% of these women considered that it had affected their day-to-day activities. Mean severity of the backache, rated on a 100 mm visual analogue scale, was 39.4. Östgaard & Anderson (1992) found similar severity ratings of backache in their sample, with an average of 3.2 on a 10 cm visual analogue scale. Average pain severity before and during pregnancy in this same cohort (surveyed earlier using the same instruments) had been 0.99 and 4.4 respectively (Östgaard & Anderson 1991). Serious postpartum backache was reported in this study by 7% of women at 12–18 months, similar to the Boston study (Groves et al 1994), in which 8% reported severe back pain at this time.

Although backache is common following childbirth and can be persistent and affect daily life, studies have found medical consultation rates to be low (MacArthur et al 1991, Bick & MacArthur 1995, Brown & Lumley 1998). It should also be noted that general population-based epidemiological studies have found prevalence estimates of back pain to be high, 14–30% in studies asking about pain on that day and 30–40% in those asking about pain in the last month (CSAG 1995). It is difficult to assess the extent of additional back pain that is attributable to childbirth.

## Risk factors

A *previous history of back pain* is an important risk factor for postnatal backache and some studies have also found a relationship with physically demanding work. Östgaard & Anderson (1992), in the cohort study described earlier, found a significant association with back pain before pregnancy; sick leave for back pain during pregnancy; and physically heavy work (the researchers were not able to determine if the effect was from work before, during or after the pregnancy). Breen et al (1994), in the Boston study, also found a history of back pain to be predictive of postpartum back pain, but only if there had also been back pain during pregnancy: Turgut et al (1998), in Turkey, followed 88 women who had back pain during pregnancy to 6 months postpartum and found that a history of pre-pregnancy back pain was a significant predictor of pain at 6 months. They found no relationship with heavy work before pregnancy but this was based on small numbers.

Breen et al (1994), in the Boston study, found *younger maternal age* and *greater maternal weight* to be predictors of postpartum backache, and Brown & Lumley (1998) found an association with heavier infant birthweight. Glazener et al (1995) found a significant association with *mode of delivery*, backache more likely after instrumental and caesarean deliveries. Brown & Lumley (1998) found proportionally more backache reported as a problem following these types of births but the difference was not statistically significant. MacArthur et al (1991) found an association with *ethnic group*, Asian women being much more likely to report backache as well as other musculoskeletal symptoms, although this may be due to cultural differences in the reporting of morbidity (MacArthur et al 1993). Loughnan et al (2002), based on data from a randomised controlled trial (RCT) of epidural versus meperidine for labour analgesia (see below), found that being non-Caucasian was an independent predictor of new backache at 6 months postpartum. Exact ethnic group was not recorded but the authors state that the hospital catchment population is 25% Asian.

The possibility of an association between *epidural analgesia* and postpartum backache has been investigated in several observational studies, some finding an association (MacArthur et al 1990, Russell et al 1993, MacLeod et al 1995, Brown & Lumley 1998), others not (Breen et al 1994, Macarthur et al 1995, Russell et al 1996). The first study on this found that 18.9% of women reported *new* backache occurring within 3 months of delivery and lasting for over 6 weeks following epidural for analgesia, compared with 10.5% of those without (MacArthur et al 1990). The suggested mechanism was through stressed postures in labour, affected by the hormone relaxin and exacerbated when discomfort feedback is inhibited by epidural block. Russell et al (1993), in a similar study at St Thomas' Hospital, London, of 612 primiparous women who received an epidural and 403 who did not, found a similar size epidural excess of new backache (17.8% vs 11.7%).

In the Boston study (Breen et al 1994) of backache at 1–2 months postpartum, epidural use was not associated with backache, either generally or with new symptoms. In a small Canadian study (Macarthur et al 1995), 164 women who had an epidural and 165 who had not were interviewed at 1 and 7 days and 6 weeks after delivery. After excluding women who had had pregnancy backache, the only difference in new postpartum backache that reached statistical significance was on day 1 (52% epidural vs 39% non-epidural), although there was a non-significant twofold epidural excess at 6 weeks (15% vs 7%). Among those followed up at 1 year, 10% had backache in the epidural and 14% in the non-epidural groups (Macarthur et al 1997).

A second study from St Thomas' Hospital, London (Russell et al 1996), compared women who requested an epidural, randomised to either a traditional (n = 157) or a mobile technique (n = 162), and a third group (n = 131) with no epidural, recruited by taking the next parity-matched delivery in the birth register. A postal questionnaire at 3 months postpartum found backache reported by 39% of the traditional group, 30% of the mobile group and 30.5% of the group with no epidural, and new backache was reported by 6.4%, 8.6% and 6.9% respectively. Like the Canadian study, since the differences were not statistically significant, the authors concluded that women could be reassured that epidurals are not associated with postpartum backache. However, both studies were small with insufficient power to detect the size of difference found in the earlier studies.

In general, the observational studies which showed no backache excess were in hospitals using a lower concentration of local anaesthetic together with an opiate, which produces less dense motor block, often allowing ambulation. A recent RCT of traditional versus two types of low-dose 'mobile' epidural techniques assessed long-term backache as an outcome (COMET Study Group 2003). This showed no significant difference in backache starting within 6 weeks of the birth and lasting longer than 3 months in either of the mobile techniques, although there was proportionally less backache in the combined-spinal than the traditional epidural group (43% vs 50%).

There have now been numerous RCTs designed to examine various possible effects of epidural versus no epidural labours, two of which have assessed backache as an outcome measure (Amin-Samuah et al 2005). Loughnan et al (2000, 2002) randomised 611 nulliparous women, of whom

249 were allocated to receive meperidine and 259 to receive epidural, and returned a 6-month questionnaire about long-term backache. The intention-to-treat comparisons showed no significant difference in any backache present at 6 months (prevalence 48% and 50% respectively) or in new backache (Loughnan et al 2002). However, there was substantial treatment cross-over, with 57% of those randomised to the meperidine group actually having an epidural, and 15% of those randomised to epidural not having one (Loughnan et al 2000). In the smaller trial by Howell et al (2001, 2002) 184 nulliparous women were randomised to epidural and 184 to no epidural, of whom 151 and 155 respectively were followed to a median of 26 months postpartum. Again, no significant differences in backache between trial groups were found. Cross-over in this trial was less, but still 28% of those randomised to no epidural had one and 33% of those randomised to epidural did not have one.

As shown above, most of the studies investigating the relationship between epidurals and backache have been observational, and since we know that women who receive epidurals generally have less straightforward labours and deliveries, these differences may account for the association. Findings from well-conducted RCTs can generally provide conclusive evidence but because epidurals provide superior pain relief than other methods, many of the women randomised to receive no epidural are likely to end up having one. It is more difficult to interpret results of RCTs where there is substantial treatment cross-over, since this will dilute any possible effect of an intervention, although a large trial would still show a large difference. The likely conclusion, therefore, on whether epidural is a risk factor for longer term postpartum backache is that if it is, any effect is likely to be relatively small.

## Management

There are no studies on the management of postpartum back pain. The evidence presented here, therefore, is based mainly on clinical guidelines prepared for the primary management of acute low back pain in the general population, first published by the Royal College of General Practitioners in 1996 and updated in 1999 (RCGP 1999). These guidelines build on a report of back pain by the Clinical Standards Advisory Group (1995), who advise the UK government, and on the review which formed the basis of the US guidelines on back pain (AHCPR 1994). A subsequent systematic review on low back pain and sciatica in the BMJ Clinical Evidence series is also drawn on (van Tulder 1999). The RCGP guideline mainly refers to acute back pain but the Clinical Evidence review separately specifies evidence on chronic back pain, which is defined as persisting for 12 weeks or more.

The CSAG report stressed the importance of primary management of backache occurring within the first 6 weeks of onset, since once chronic pain is established any form of treatment has a lower chance of success (CSAG 1995). This is of particular relevance for postnatal management, since consultation rates for postpartum backache are low (MacArthur et al 1991, Bick &

MacArthur 1995, Brown & Lumley 1998), highlighting the need to specifically ask women about symptoms to ensure prompt identification and management.

The guidelines present evidence relating to an assessment of the type of backache, including the role of psychological factors, and on management, the latter comprising symptomatic measures (drug therapy, bed rest, advice on staying active) and physical therapies (manipulation and back exercise).

## Assessment

Assessment of the type of backache as simple or non-specific is first required to exclude possible serious spinal pathology and to distinguish nerve root pain or sciatica, for which management is slightly different. There is now a great deal of evidence, with consistent findings from several prospective cohort studies, that psychosocial factors are particularly important in relation to chronic low back pain, that they influence a patient's response to treatment and rehabilitation and that they are important at a much earlier stage than previously believed (RCGP 1999).

## Drugs, bedrest, advice to stay active

Management options for back pain have been extensively investigated with good-quality evidence. In terms of *drug therapy*, analgesics (paracetamol, paracetamol–weak opioid compounds and NSAIDs) are all effective in reducing acute back pain. Comparisons between paracetamol and paracetamol–weak opioid compounds with NSAIDs are inconsistent, but the RCGP guidelines recommend paracetamol as first-line drug therapy, followed by NSAIDs, then paracetamol–weak opioid compounds (such as codydramol or coproxamol), probably because of side-effects of the various preparations. RCTs examining a variety of muscle relaxants show that these are effective in reducing acute low back pain but there are side-effects of drowsiness and dizziness and a risk of dependency (RCGP 1999, van Tulder 1999). For chronic back pain evidence suggests that analgesics and NSAIDs are both likely to be of benefit, but there is no evidence on muscle relaxants (van Tulder 1999).

The effectiveness of *bed rest* has been investigated in numerous RCTs, which consistently show that this is not an effective treatment option, with adverse effects of prolonged bed rest, such as joint stiffness and debilitation (RCGP 1999, van Tulder 1999). RCTs of *advice to stay active* are consistent in showing benefits of this in terms of faster rates of recovery, less pain, less sick leave and less chronic disability, compared with bed rest or with usual care. There are no studies, of an acceptable quality, of the effects of either bed rest or advice to stay active on chronic back pain.

## Physical therapies

Physical therapies, both manipulation and back exercises, have been examined in a large number of RCTs, although many are of poor quality. For *manipulation* the RCGP guidelines (1999) and the systematic review by van Tulder (1999) conclude that there are inconsistencies in the results. The RCGP report notes, however, that more of the trials report positive than negative results of manipulation in the short-term improvement in pain and activity. Evidence on the effect of spinal manipulation on chronic back pain is conflicting. In relation to *back exercises*, RCTs show that it is doubtful that these produce clinically significant improvement in acute low back pain. For chronic pain, however, there is some evidence that exercise programmes can improve pain and functional levels, compared to conservative or a variety of inactive treatments (e.g. hot packs, TENS).

## SUMMARY OF THE EVIDENCE USED IN THIS GUIDELINE

- Numerous large prospective studies have shown that backache is a common postpartum problem, occurring in 20–50% of women. Severe back pain occurs in just under 10%. Backache after childbirth often persists, but since prevalence is also high in the general population, the size of excess attributable to childbirth is difficult to assess.
- The most important risk factor for postpartum backache is a previous history of backache. Some studies have found a variety of other risk factors. Evidence on whether backache is associated with epidural analgesia is still not conclusive, although if there is any effect it is likely to be small.
- There is no specific evidence relating to postnatal management. Evidence from randomised controlled trials of the management of acute low back pain among the general population has shown that analgesics and advice to stay active are beneficial, but bed rest is ineffective. Psychological factors have an effect on treatment response.

## WHAT TO DO

### Initial assessment

The clinical history should take account of:

- The description of the symptom (for example, is it mostly in the back or does it refer to one or both legs, or is there any numbness or paraesthesia?) and its duration.
- Any complicating psychosocial factors.
- Any history of trauma.

Following the RCGP guidelines (1999), this will enable assessment of the backache as:

- Simple backache
- Nerve root pain (sciatica)
- Possible serious spinal pathology.

## Symptoms which require urgent action

- Possible serious spinal pathology.
- Onset associated with trauma.
- Severe pain, especially if affecting daily activities.

## General advice

- Reassure that backache is common after childbirth and that there are various successful management options available.
- The woman may benefit from practical advice on correct posture when handling, lifting and feeding the infant. The Association of Chartered Physiotherapists provides a simple leaflet which may be helpful, if available locally. Work through the literature with the woman to ensure that she understands it.

## Management of simple backache

- Analgesia (paracetamol as first-line) should be taken on a regular basis to control pain.
- If paracetamol is not providing adequate pain relief, referral should be made for more powerful analgesia (NSAIDs or paracetamol–weak opioid compounds), ensuring advice is given about possible adverse side-effects, such as constipation (urgent action).
- Advise the woman to continue with her normal activity as much as possible.
- Depending on symptom severity, if there is no significant improvement after a week or two, the woman should be referred (non-urgent action) since treatment within 6 weeks of onset is recommended (CSAG 1995).
- If the symptoms have not worsened advise the woman to continue with normal activity, and reduce the amount of analgesia she is taking.
- Psychological management is important, for example encouraging the woman to have a positive attitude to activity and childcare. Back pain may be an indicator of psychological distress and depressive symptoms. (If this is suspected refer to the guideline on Depression and Other Psychological Problems (Chapter 7)).

# SUMMARY GUIDELINE

## Backache

### Initial assessment

- Ask about duration and description of problem
- Ask about any complicating psychosocial factors
- Ask about history of trauma

### Urgent action is required if:

- Possible serious spinal pathology
- Onset associated with trauma
- Severe pain, especially affecting daily activities

## What to do

### Simple postpartum backache

- Analgesia (paracetamol as first-line) should be taken on a regular basis
- If paracetamol is not satisfactory refer for more powerful analgesia (urgent action)
- Advise to continue with normal activity
- If no significant improvement, refer as treatment within six weeks of onset is recommended (non-urgent action)
- Psychological management should include the encouragement of a positive attitude to activity and childcare

### General advice

- Reassure that backache is common after childbirth and there are various successful management options available. It will improve with simple analgesia and normal activity which will reduce the risk of problem becoming chronic
- Give the woman a copy of the leaflet from the Association of Chartered Physiotherapists (if available)
- Advise on correct posture when handling, lifting and feeding the infant

# References

Agency for Health Care Policy and Research (AHCPR) 1994 Management guidelines for acute low back pain. Agency for Health Care Policy and Research, US Department of Health and Human Services, Rockville, Maryland

Amin-Samuah M, Smyth R, Howell C 2005 Epidural versus non-epidural or no analgesia in labour. Cochrane Database of Systematic Reviews, Issue 4

Berg G, Hammar M, Moller-Nielsen J et al 1988 Low back pain during pregnancy. Obstet Gynecol 71(1): 71-75

Bick D, MacArthur C 1995 The extent, severity and effect of health problems after childbirth. Br J Midwif 3(1): 27-31

Breen T, Ransil B, Groves P et al 1994 Factors associated with back pain after childbirth. Anesthesiology 81(1): 29-34

Brown S, Lumley J 1998 Maternal health after childbirth: results of an Australian population based survey. Br J Obstet Gynaecol 105: 156-161

Clinical Standards Advisory Group (CSAG) 1995 Back pain. Chaired by Professor Michael Rosen. HMSO, London

COMET Study Group 2003 Comparative Mobile Epidural Trial: long-term outcomes. Society for Obstetric Anaesthesia and Perinatology. Anesthesiology 93(suppl): A75

Fast A, Shapiro D, Ducommun E et al 1987 Low back pain during pregnancy. Spine 12: 368-371

Garcia J, Redshaw M, Fitzsimons B et al 1998 First Class Delivery. A national survey of women's views of maternity care. Audit Commission Publications, Abingdon, Oxford.

Glazener C, Abdalla M, Russell I et al 1993 Postnatal care: a survey of patients' experiences. Br J Midwif 1(2): 67-74

Glazener C, Abdalla M, Stoud P et al 1995 Postnatal maternal morbidity: extent, causes, prevention and treatment. Br J Obstet Gynaecol 102(4): 282-287

Groves P, Breen T, Ransil B et al 1994 Natural history of post partum back pain and its relationship with epidural anesthesia. Anesthesiology 81(3A): A1167

Howell C, Kidd C, Roberts W et al 2001 A randomised controlled trial of epidural compared with non-epidural analgesia in labour. Br J Obstet Gynaecol 108: 27-33

Howell C, Dean T, Lucking L et al 2002 Randomised study of long term outcome after epidural versus non-epidural analgesia in labour. BMJ 325: 357-361

Loughnan B, Carli F, Romney M et al 2000 Randomized controlled comparison of epidural bupivacaine *versus* pethidine for analgesia in labour. Br J Anaesth 84: 715-719

Loughnan B, Carli F, Romney M et al 2002 Epidural analgesia and backache: a randomized controlled comparison with intramuscular meperidine for analgesia during labour. Br J Anaesth 89: 466-472

Macarthur A, MacArthur C, Weeks S 1995 Epidural anaesthesia and low back pain after delivery: a prospective cohort study. BMJ 311: 1336-1339

Macarthur A, MacArthur C, Weeks S 1997 Is epidural anesthesia in labor associated with chronic low back pain? A prospective cohort study. Anesth Analg 85: 1066-1070

MacArthur C, Lewis M, Knox E et al 1990 Epidural anaesthesia and long term backache after childbirth. BMJ 301: 9-12

MacArthur C, Lewis M, Knox E 1991 Health after childbirth. HMSO, London

MacArthur C, Lewis M, Knox E 1993 Comparison of long-term health problems following childbirth in Asian and Caucasian women. Br J Gen Pract 42: 519-522

MacLennan A, Nicholson R, Green R et al 1986 Serum relaxin and pelvic pain of pregnancy. Lancet ii: 243-245

MacLeod J, Macintyre C, McClure J et al 1995 Backache and epidural analgesia. Int J Obstet Anesth 4: 21-25

Östgaard H, Anderson G 1991 Previous back pain and risk of developing back pain in a future pregnancy. Spine 16(4): 432-436

Östgaard H, Anderson G 1992 Postpartum low-back pain. Spine 17: 53-55

Royal College of General Practitioners (RCGP) 1999 Clinical guidelines for the management of acute low back pain. RCGP Press, London

Russell R, Groves P, Taub N et al 1993 Assessing long term backache after childbirth. BMJ 306: 1299-1303

Russell R, Dundas R, Raynolds F 1996 Long term backache after childbirth: prospective search for causative factors. BMJ 312: 1384-1388

Saurel-Cubizolles M-J, Romito P, Lelong N et al 2000 Women's health after childbirth: a longitudinal study in France and Italy. Br J Obstet Gynaecol 107: 1202-1209

Turgut F, Turgut M, Çetinsahin M 1998 A prospective study of persistent back pain after pregnancy. Eur J Obst Gynecol Reprod Biol 80: 45-48

van Tulder M 1999 Low back pain and sciatica. Clinical Evidence (BMJ) 2: 406-422

# Chapter 10

# Headache

## INTRODUCTION

The two types of headache commonly reported among the general population are tension headache and migraine, both of which are more frequent among women, possibly related to hormonal factors (Rasmussen 1993). According to the *International Classification of Headache Disorders* (ICHD) (International Headache Society 2004), primary headaches can be categorised as migraine, tension-type headache, cluster headache and other trigeminal autonomic cephalalgias, and other primary headaches. A tension-type headache is the most common form of primary headache. Symptoms are usually bilateral and include pressing or tightening feelings of mild or moderate intensity, with no nausea or vomiting, and not aggravated by routine physical activity. Phonophobia or photophobia is possible, but not both. A migraine headache without aura (the commonest subtype of migraine) tends to be unilateral and pulsating, of moderate to severe intensity, is aggravated by routine physical activity and is accompanied by at least two symptoms of nausea, vomiting, photophobia and phonophobia (International Headache Society 2004). Onset in women is often related to menstruation. Whether these types of headaches are more common among postpartum than non-postpartum women is not known, since there are no comparative studies. There is some information, however, about headaches in the postnatal period from studies of health problems in postpartum populations. In addition, there are some conditions which are more common among postnatal women and which can present with, or result in, headaches.

These are postdural puncture headaches following spinal or epidural anaesthesia; headache associated with postpartum hypertension, pre-eclampsia or eclampsia; and subarachnoid haemorrhage. All of these are reviewed in this guideline.

## POSTPARTUM 'SIMPLE' HEADACHE

### Frequency of occurrence and risk factors

Studies that have examined the occurrence of headaches early after childbirth suggest that these are experienced by 20–40% of women on one or more days during the first week (Grove 1973, Pitt 1973, Stein 1981, Stein et al 1984). Garcia & Marchant (1993), in an observational study of postnatal health at 8 weeks among 90 women, found that 23% had experienced headaches at some time since the birth. Longer term studies in postpartum populations have also found frequent headaches to be common. In one large observational study of a variety of health problems after childbirth, 419 (4%) of 11,701 women reported frequent headaches which had begun for the first time within 3 months of the delivery and lasted for over 6 weeks, and a further 5% reported similar frequent headaches which they had also had sometime before. The corresponding proportions reporting migraine were 1% and 6%, indicating that migraine was less likely to be a *new* postpartum problem (MacArthur et al 1991). Glazener et al (1995), in a longitudinal study, examined maternal postnatal morbidity in over 1200 women, who comprised a 20% random sample of deliveries in the Grampian region of Scotland between June 1990 and May 1991. All women were given a questionnaire whilst on the postnatal ward, a postal questionnaire at 8 weeks, and half were sent another questionnaire 12–18 months after the birth. Headaches of any duration, including new and recurrent symptoms, were reported by 14% of women whilst in hospital, by 22% between then and 8 weeks and by 15% after this. A large cluster randomised controlled trial (RCT) of a new model of midwifery-led postnatal care, which focused on the identification and management of common health problems up to 12 weeks after the birth, included the same health problems in a questionnaire completed by women 12 months after the birth. At 12 months headaches were reported by 26% of women overall, with no difference in symptoms between the intervention and control groups (MacArthur et al 2003). As with the study by Glazener et al (1995), women were not asked to distinguish between new and ongoing symptoms.

A longitudinal survey of Italian and French women's health after childbirth found that headache prevalence had increased at 12 months postpartum compared with at 5 months: 45% of Italian women reported headaches at 12 months compared with 22% at 5 months, and 38% of French women had headaches at 12 months compared with 21% at 5 months (Saurel-Cubizolles et al 2000). Reasons for this were not postulated.

An additional finding of MacArthur et al (1991) was that some headaches, occurring with musculoskeletal symptoms, were more likely to start during the first postnatal week and were associated with epidural analgesia for pain relief. Frequent headaches or migraine in women without musculoskeletal symptoms were associated with younger age, multiparity and lower social class, and not with epidural analgesia, and were probably related more to factors within the social environment than to the delivery. Headaches in the first postpartum week were found to be associated with psychological morbidity by Stein et al (1984). In this study, the occurrence of headache was documented daily among 71 women who were asked to complete a self-rating questionnaire, which also included questions on the presence of tension, depression and feelings of weepiness. Women who developed a headache on at least one day were more depressed and had more tension than those who did not. Details of the self-rating schedule were not described, thus its validity cannot be assessed.

## Management

Studies of headache after hospital discharge were all investigating postnatal health more generally, and relied on self-reports of headaches, without obtaining detailed classificatory information of the sort used to distinguish different types of headache as in the ICHD (2004). It is likely, however, that most postpartum headaches are tension headaches, the next most common being migraine, most of which will be reported by women who have a previous history of this. The main role of the midwife is to assess the headache in order to refer those that are due to other causes. The management of tension headaches and migraine is the same as for general population groups (Barrett 1996), but taking care that any analgesia is appropriate for breastfeeding mothers.

## POSTDURAL PUNCTURE HEADACHE

### Definition

A postdural puncture headache (PDPH) may occur following the administration of an epidural or spinal needle for pain relief in labour or for caesarean section. In the case of spinal anaesthesia the dura is punctured deliberately, whilst an accidental dural puncture occurs occasionally during the insertion of the epidural needle. The diagnosis of an accidental dural puncture is usually made by the anaesthetist during insertion of the epidural, when cerebrospinal fluid (CSF) is observed, but some cases are diagnosed retrospectively following the onset of headache in the puerperium.

Headache after dural puncture results from a loss of CSF, with subsequent traction on the meninges, and has several typical presenting characteristics. The most significant is its postural nature; the headache gets dramatically worse when the patient moves from the supine to the upright position, and conversely is markedly diminished or relieved totally when lying down (Katz & Aidinis 1980). The associated symptoms of neck stiffness, visual disturbances, vomiting and auditory effects may also be reported, but are more common with severe PDPH (Lybecker et al 1995, Banks et al 2001).

## Frequency of occurrence and risk factors

The incidence of accidental dural puncture during epidural is now between about 0.18% and 3.6%, although it had been higher than this when epidural was first used in routine obstetric practice (Gleeson & Reynolds 1998). Where this type of puncture does occur, however, the relatively large diameter of the epidural needle means that loss of CSF is likely and the incidence of PDPH is high. This high incidence is also attributed to bearing down in the second stage of labour which may exacerbate CSF leakage; to decreased intra-abdominal pressure following delivery which causes the epidural veins to collapse; and to rapid loss of fluid from blood loss, diuresis and lactation (Gutsche 1990). In a case-note analysis of 20 years of women with accidental puncture in one maternity unit, the incidence of typical PDPH was 86% (Stride & Cooper 1993). The majority of the women (69%) in this series developed their headache within the first 2 days of delivery, although it could also appear up to 6 days after (Stride & Cooper 1993).

A lower incidence of PDPH was reported in a large UK survey of outcomes following anaesthetic interventions. The National Obstetric Anaesthetic Database (NOAD) was established in the UK in 1998, to support collection of national data on obstetric analgesia and anaesthesia. Data for the first year aimed to determine the incidence, characteristics, contributing factors and management of postpartum headaches associated with anaesthetic interventions (Chan et al 2003). Data were requested from all members of the Obstetric Anaesthetists Association in the UK in 1999, who were asked to provide complete data for at least 1 month continuously for their unit on anaesthetic activity and number of headaches reported. Symptoms were to have lasted for more than 6 hours, unrelieved by mild analgesics. Data were supported with an anonymous individual case record for each incident reported. Data were collected on 65,348 women from 93 obstetric units, 38,271 (59%) of whom had an epidural; 16,844 (26%) had a spinal; 4926 (8%) had a combined spinal-epidural (CSE); 4203 (6%) had a general anaesthetic (GA); 939 (1%) had a GA and regional block; and 165 (0.2%) had a combination of regional techniques. The incidence of headache ranged from 1.1% to 1.9% between all anaesthetic techniques, which increased to 10.9% for multiple regional anaesthetics. Individual case records were returned for 1101 women, 975 of whom had an anaesthetic intervention. Headaches in the 975 women were divided into cases where a PDPH had been diagnosed (404, 41%) and non-PDPH (571, 59%) based on information provided. As data were only collected on women who were inpatients, and given the potential for incomplete data collection, the incidence of PDPH may have been higher. Other outcomes of interest reported in the survey are described later in this chapter.

Most PDPHs are of relatively short duration, lasting for several days (Crawford 1972). In the study described earlier of health problems after child-birth among 11,701 women, however, 74 were recorded as having an accidental dural puncture and 23% of these reported frequent headaches or migraine lasting for longer than 6 weeks. Information on whether these headaches were of a postural nature was not obtained, although some women also reported neckache or visual or auditory disturbances (MacArthur et al 1993).

Much smaller diameter needles are used for spinal than for epidural analgesia, so that although a spinal always punctures the dura, with current types of spinal needles (see below), similar proportions of PDPHs occur after each procedure. Spinal anaesthesia has been used for a variety of surgical and investigative interventions for 100 years or so, but the early incidence of PDPH was high. In a classic study from the USA of a general series of 10,098 spinals, it was noted that obstetric patients had the highest headache rates (Vandam & Dripps 1956). In 1979, Crawford reported a PDPH rate of 16% in an obstetric unit that was a specialist centre for regional blocks (Crawford 1979). Spinal needles of smaller diameter and designs that spread rather than cut the dural fibres have since become popular and have made a significant impact on the incidence of postspinal headache (Turnbull & Shepherd 2003). A general population-based meta-analysis, which found rates of all headaches ranging from 1% to almost 30%, and rates of severe headaches from none to 12%, concluded that smaller and non-cutting needles were associated with the lowest rates (Halpern & Preston 1994). A randomised controlled trial of spinal anaesthesia for caesarean section compared a 25 gauge diamond-tipped needle with a 24 gauge non-cutting Sprotte needle (Cesarini et al 1990). The trial planned to recruit 100 women to each group but was stopped at 55, when a PDPH rate of 14.5% was shown in the former group, compared with none in the Sprotte group. Other obstetric studies comparing different needles have had similar findings (e.g. Shutt et al 1992). In addition to needle size, the direction of insertion of the needle has also been considered. A meta-analysis based on general population data was undertaken to determine if bevel direction during lumbar puncture would influence the incidence of PDPH (Richman et al 2006). The results indicated that use of a cutting needle with insertion in a parallel/longitudinal fashion may significantly reduce the incidence of PDPH, although reasons for the decrease were unclear.

Most maternity units now report incidence rates of severe headaches requiring blood patch of about 1% or less (Hopkinson et al 1997, Madej et al 1993). Mild headaches have been documented in up to 10% (Hopkinson et al 1997), but the extent to which these might be attributed to the spinal is not known since, as described earlier, headaches in the first few days after birth are generally quite common. Data from the NOAD survey described earlier (Chan et al 2003) found that of the 404 women who had a diagnosed PDPH, severe headaches were reported by 202 (50%), a much higher proportion than reported in the non-PDPH group (p < 0.0001), and 305 (75%) of these women reported that the headache limited their daily activity (p < 0.0001).

Epidural analgesia remains a common intervention in labour, with most units now offering lower-dose infusions which enable women to mobilise. In a recent Cochrane systematic review of CSE with epidural analgesia in labour which included data from 14 trials (2047 women), a total of 25 outcomes were analysed (Hughes et al 2003). No difference was found between CSE and epidural techniques with regard to the incidence of PDPH or blood patch (see below), hypotension, urinary retention, mode of delivery or admission of the baby to the neonatal unit.

Another Cochrane review compared outcomes following spinal or epidural for caesarean section (Ng et al 2004). Ten trials were included in the review, which provided data on a total of 751 women. The reviewers could not draw any conclusion about intraoperative side-effects and postoperative complications, such as PDPH, due to small numbers reported.

## Management

Since many women are now discharged from hospital before a PDPH is likely to develop, it is important that the midwife is able to identify this type of headache (Cooper 1999), and if the headache is severe, referral must be made to the appropriate healthcare professional, according to local policy. In the case of a known accidental dural puncture the anaesthetist may have already instituted prophylactic measures or begun treatment if symptoms were severe.

A clinical review of the treatment of PDPH in the general population notes that conservative treatment is recommended in the first instance, which includes simple analgesics (e.g. paracetamol), bed rest and hydration. Bed rest seems to alleviate symptoms, although this has not been found to be effective in preventing a headache occurring (McSwiney & Phillips 1995). An evaluation of the literature (including clinical studies, letters, abstracts and case reports) on the pharmacological management of PDPH in general populations concluded that intravenous and oral caffeine are effective treatments, and at least non-invasive, but that more clinical studies are required to properly evaluate other pharmacotherapies. In the meantime, the authors suggest that therapy be guided by clinical judgement (Choi et al 1996).

Epidural blood patch is now considered by many obstetric anaesthetists to be an effective treatment for severe PDPH after accidental puncture or spinal anaesthesia, but this is unsupported by evidence of effectiveness from RCTs. A blood patch involves injecting 10–20 ml of the woman's blood into the epidural space around the site of the dural puncture; the blood coagulates and seals the leak of CSF. A second blood patch is sometimes given in the event of failure. A success rate of over 90% has been reported in some observational studies, although others report permanent symptom relief in about two-thirds (Stride & Cooper 1993, Taivainen et al 1993).

There is controversy about the use of blood patching as a prophylactic measure where accidental dural puncture is known to have occurred (Cooper 1999). Berger et al (1998), in a survey of the management of accidental dural puncture during labour in 36 centres in North America, found that almost half used prophylactic blood patching. In the NOAD survey (Chan et al 2003), 242 (60%) of the 404 women with a diagnosed PDPH received a blood patch, with 101 (42%) performed within 2 days of the onset of symptoms and almost all (91%) performed within 8 days. Data on outcome following blood patch were not provided. A Cochrane library systematic review of epidural blood patching for prevention and treatment of PDPH (Sudlow & Warlow 2001) included three trials with data from 77 general population patients. Methodological details were generally incomplete. Although the results of the analyses suggested that both prophylactic and therapeutic epidural blood patching may be of benefit, the very small number of patients and outcome events, as well as uncertainties about trial methodology, precluded reliable assessments of the potential benefits and harms of blood patching. Further, adequately powered randomised trials (including at least a few hundred patients) are required before reliable conclusions can be drawn about the effectiveness of epidural blood patching.

## HYPERTENSIVE DISORDERS

Much has been written on the hypertensive disorders of pregnancy and there are various differing definitions. It is included in this guideline because headache can be one of its manifestations and because these disorders can occur in the postpartum period.

## Hypertension

Pregnancy-induced hypertension (PIH) is commonly reported and was defined in a clinical review of the hypertensive disorders of pregnancy as the recording of a blood pressure of 140/90 mmHg or more on two occasions 4 or more hours apart after the 20th week of pregnancy, in a previously normotensive woman (Broughton Pipkin 1995). The hypertensive disorders of pregnancy comprise a spectrum of conditions that are usually classified into four categories: (i) gestational hypertension, a rise in blood pressure during the second half of pregnancy; (ii) pre-eclampsia, usually hypertension with proteinuria (protein in urine) during the second half of pregnancy; (iii) chronic hypertension, a rise in blood pressure prior to pregnancy or before 20 weeks' gestation and (iv) pre-eclampsia superimposed on chronic hypertension (Gifford et al 2000).

### Frequency of occurrence

Around 10% of women will have raised blood pressure at some point before delivery (Meher & Duley 2006), and pre-eclampsia complicates around 2–8%

of pregnancies (WHO 1988). The aetiology of hypertension remains unknown. Walters et al (1986) measured the blood pressure of 136 previously normotensive women in the morning and afternoon for 5 days following normal delivery. Both systolic and diastolic blood pressure rose for the first 4 days, leading the authors to conclude that a rise in blood pressure during this period seems to represent a general phenomenon. In the background to a Cochrane systematic review of prevention and management of postpartum hypertension, postpartum blood pressure was reported to be highest at around 6 days after birth (Magee & Sadeghi 2005), following which measures will fall. This pattern of blood pressure is thought to result from mobilisation, from the extravascular to the intravascular space, of the 6–8 litres of total body water and the 950 mEq of total body sodium accumulated during pregnancy (Magee & Sadeghi 2005). Other studies have examined the postnatal duration of hypertension among women who have already presented with PIH or pre-eclampsia. Ferrazzani et al (1994) studied 269 women with PIH (n = 159) or pre-eclampsia (n = 110) and monitored their postpartum blood pressure daily after delivery until a diastolic blood pressure of ≤110 mmHg was reached. The time taken for this ranged from 0 to 10 days among the PIH women and from 0 to 23 days among those with pre-eclampsia. How long it took for women to become 'normotensive' (diastolic ≤80 mmHg), however, was not reported.

The true prevalence of postpartum hypertension is difficult to ascertain, but the importance of monitoring women after birth was highlighted by the *Confidential enquiries into maternal deaths in the United Kingdom* (Lewis & Drife 2004) in which roughly 10% of maternal deaths due to a hypertensive disorder occurred in the postpartum period. The inadequate management of hypertension was highlighted. Women who have antenatal pre-eclampsia appear to have a higher risk of postpartum hypertension (Tan & de Swiet 2002).

In addition to headache, other symptoms that sometimes accompany a rise in blood pressure include photophobia, visual disturbances, vomiting or epigastric discomfort, although these are not as likely to occur in less severe cases.

## Management

The aim of the Cochrane systematic review of prevention and treatment of postpartum hypertension was to assess the relative benefits and risks of interventions (Magee & Sadeghi 2005).

Six trials were included in the review. With regard to *prevention*, three trials (315 women; six comparisons) compared furosemide or nifedipine capsules with placebo/no therapy; however, there were insufficient data to enable conclusions about possible benefits and risks of these management strategies to be drawn. Most outcomes included data from only one trial. With regard to *treatment*, in two trials (106 women; three comparisons), oral timolol or hydralazine was compared with oral methyldopa for treatment of mild to moderate postpartum hypertension. In one trial (38 women; one comparison), oral hydralazine plus sublingual nifedipine was compared with sublingual nifedipine for treatment of severe postpartum hypertension. The need for additional antihypertensive therapy did not differ between groups (relative ratio (RR) 4.24, 95% confidence interval (CI) 0.96–18.84). The reviewers concluded that there are no reliable data to guide management of women who are hypertensive postpartum or at increased risk of developing hypertension, and management decisions should be based on clinical judgement. Future studies of prevention or treatment of postpartum hypertension should include information about use of postpartum analgesics and outcomes of severe maternal hypertension; breastfeeding; hospital length of stay; and maternal satisfaction with care.

## Postpartum pre-eclampsia and eclampsia

Pre-eclampsia is considered to occur when PIH is associated with significant proteinurea (300 mg/l in 24h) (Davey & MacGillivray 1988). The precise relationship between PIH and pre-eclampsia, however, is still unclear. The most common definition of *eclampsia* is convulsions, plus the usual signs and symptoms of pre-eclampsia, where other causes of convulsion have been excluded (Douglas & Redman 1994). Fourteen maternal deaths due to eclampsia or pre-eclampsia were reported in the UK between 2000 and 2002 (Lewis & Drife 2004), seven of which occurred after the birth.

### Frequency of occurrence

There is some variation in the reported incidence of postpartum pre-eclampsia and eclampsia. One possible explanation for this may be the variation in the definition used, and the duration of the period studied. Douglas & Redman (1994) undertook a prospective survey of all hospitals with a consultant obstetric unit as well as questionnaires to GPs, to document the incidence of eclampsia in the UK in 1992. The precise definition of eclampsia used in the survey was the occurrence of convulsions during pregnancy, labour or within 10 postpartum days, together with at least two of the following within 24 hours of the convulsion: hypertension, proteinuria, thrombocytopenia or raised plasma aspartate transaminase concentration. The number of cases identified was 383, an incidence of 4.9 per 10,000 maternities, and 1 in 50 of the women died. Most (85%) women had been seen by a doctor or midwife in the preceding week, 43% of whom had not had hypertension with proteinuria, and some (11%) had had neither of these signs. Antecedent symptoms had been experienced by 59% of the eclamptic women, 50% had headaches, 19% visual disturbances and 19% epigastric pain. Among all the women with eclampsia, 44% were found to occur in the postpartum period. The proportion of postpartum cases occurring without hypertension, proteinuria or antecedent symptoms is not given, but expert opinion suggests that it is unlikely to be different from the overall pattern.

Lubarsky et al (1994) undertook a 15-year (1977–1992) case-note review in one unit in the USA to investigate *late* postpartum eclampsia – convulsions which occurred between 48 hours and 4 weeks postpartum. During this period 112,500 women delivered and there was a total of 334 cases of eclampsia. Among these, 97 (29%) occurred postpartum, 54 of which were classed as late postpartum, occurring as long as 23 days after delivery, although most occurred much earlier than this. Of the 54 women with late postpartum eclampsia, 45 (83%) had prodromal symptoms: 38 (70%) reported severe headache and 17 (31%) visual disturbances, with some women reporting both symptoms. The duration of symptoms prior to convulsion was between 2 and 72 hours. The authors noted that the subjective signs and symptoms of severe and persistent occipital headache, photophobia, blurred vision or scotomata and epigastric pain can serve as a clinical warning before the onset of convulsions. The majority of late postpartum convulsions in this study occurred after hospital discharge.

Atterbury et al (1998), in a retrospective case–control study, identified 57 women from 32,762 in one unit who were subsequently readmitted with severe pre-eclampsia or eclampsia at a rate of 1.7 per 1000 maternities. Four women were excluded because of incomplete case notes and the remaining 53 (32 with pre-eclampsia and 21 with eclampsia) were matched two-to-one with 106 women who had intrapartum severe pre-eclampsia or eclampsia. Detailed information on symptoms, physical findings and laboratory assays was obtained. The case–control comparison showed that headache, visual disturbances, nausea and vomiting and malaise were reported significantly more by postpartum women on readmission than controls had reported during labour or in the immediate postpartum period. The occurrence of oedema and epigastric pain did not vary between cases and controls. In postpartum women headaches were positively correlated with systolic, diastolic and mean arterial blood pressure, but this relationship was not found in the control group. Women readmitted with symptoms were more likely to develop seizures than women in the control group.

In another study from the USA, Chames and colleagues (2002) investigated late postpartum eclampsia in a multicentre analysis of data from women who gave birth from 1996 to 2001, defining 'late' as being a seizure which occurred more than 48 hours after the birth. Data were collected from three centres on the relationship of the woman's first seizure to delivery, prodromal symptoms, neuroimaging studies, use of magnesium sulphate, antihypertensive therapy and follow-up medical care. Eighty-nine women were diagnosed with eclampsia; 29 women had a postpartum onset, 23 of whom (79%) had late onset. Twenty-one (91%) women had at least one prodromal symptom, and 12 (52%) had one or more symptoms which heralded the onset of the seizure. This included 20 (87%) women who had a headache; 10 (44%) who had visual changes; five (22%) had nausea or vomiting; and two women experienced epigastric pain. Of note is that few of the 21 women (n = 7/33%) sought care for their symptoms. Despite the study limitations, including reliance on accuracy of diagnosis coding and potential for incomplete data collection, the importance of ensuring that clinicians and women are aware of symptoms is emphasised.

In a 5-year prospective study to identify the risk of serious complications from severe pre-eclampsia and eclampsia, Tufnell and colleagues (2005) collated data on 1087 women diagnosed with severe pre-eclampsia or eclampsia from 210,631 women who gave birth in 16 maternity units in Yorkshire, UK (5.2/1000); 151 women had serious complications, including 82 who had eclamptic seizures. Of the 82 women who had eclampsia, 26 (32%) had seizures after giving birth.

## Management

Although routine antenatal screening measures, which should include testing urine for proteinuria and monitoring of the woman's blood pressure (NICE 2003), may enable the detection of women at risk of pre-eclampsia and eclampsia, it is important to note, as shown above, that eclamptic seizures can occur without antenatal indicators and after hospital postnatal discharge. Eclampsia can occur unheralded by signs and possibly even by symptoms, and certainly with only short-duration ones. Women may have an eclamptic fit despite previously having a relatively low diastolic blood pressure (Douglas & Redman 1994). Community midwives must therefore be alert to all possible warning signs and symptoms. Where a woman has hypertension and complains of a headache in the postpartum period and there are symptoms of pre-eclampsia, such as epigastric discomfort, visual disturbance, nausea or vomiting, immediate referral for assessment should be made.

A Cochrane systematic review assessed the effectiveness of magnesium sulphate and other anticonvulsants for women with pre-eclampsia either before or after delivery (Duley et al 2003a). Six trials which presented data on 11,444 women compared magnesium sulphate with placebo or no anticonvulsant. There was more than a halving in the risk of eclampsia associated with magnesium sulphate (RR 0.41, 95% CI 0.29–0.58). The risk of dying was non-significantly reduced by 46% for women allocated magnesium sulphate (RR 0.54, 95% CI 0.26–1.10), with no clear evidence of difference in effect on serious maternal morbidity (RR 1.08, 95% CI 0.89–1.32). Side-effects were more common with magnesium sulphate (24% versus 5%; RR 5.26, 95% CI 4.59–6.03). Risk of placental abruption was reduced for women who received magnesium sulphate, although there was a small increase (5%) in the risk of caesarean section. There was no overall difference in the risk of stillbirth or neonatal death. Magnesium sulphate was better than phenytoin for reducing the risk of eclampsia (two trials, 2241 women; RR 0.05, 95% CI 0.00–0.84), but with an increased risk of caesarean section (RR 1.21, 95% CI 1.05–1.41). It was also better than nimodipine (one trial, 1650 women; RR 0.33, 95% CI 0.14–0.77).

Two Cochrane systematic reviews of treatment for eclampsia compared the use of magnesium sulphate with other drugs. One review compared magnesium sulphate with diazepam (Duley & Henderson-Smart 2003b) and the other compared magnesium sulphate with phenytoin (Duley & Henderson-Smart 2003c). Both reviews concluded that magnesium sulphate was substantially more effective in reducing the recurrence of convulsions than each of the other treatments (diazepam RR 0.45, 95% CI 0.35–0.58; phenytoin RR 0.30, 95% CI 0.20–0.46).

The NICE postnatal care guideline (NICE 2006) recommends that all women have a minimum of one blood pressure recording taken and documented within 6 hours of giving birth, and that within the first 24 hours of birth, all women receive information on signs and symptoms of potentially life-threatening conditions, including pre-eclampsia/eclampsia. Signs and symptoms women should seek urgent attention for include headaches accompanied by one or more of the following: visual disturbances, vomiting, and nausea and vomiting. Further information is given in the 'What to Do' section at the end of this guideline.

## SUBARACHNOID HAEMORRHAGE

### Definition

A subarachnoid haemorrhage (SAH) is a bleed into the subarachnoid space. It often presents with a violent and unusual headache, often described as thunderclap. Case reports of non-puerperal cases have described presenting symptoms as including sudden severe headache and vomiting (Wasserberg & Barlow 1997).

### Frequency of occurrence and risk factors

In the most recent triennial report on *Confidential enquiries into maternal deaths in the UK 2000–2002* (Lewis & Drife 2004), there were more deaths from SAH than from pre-eclampsia/eclampsia; there were 21 cases of intracranial haemorrhage, 17 due to subarachnoid haemorrhage and four to intracerebral haemorrhage. These deaths were classified as 'other indirect deaths'. *Indirect* maternal deaths are defined as deaths resulting from previously existing disease or disease which develops during pregnancy which was not due to direct obstetric causes, but was aggravated by physiological effects of pregnancy (Lewis & Drife 2004). The ages of the women who died of SAH varied between 19 years and 39 years, with a mean of 32 years. In three cases the timing of bleeding in relation to stage of pregnancy was unknown. Four of the bleeds occurred antenatally, two in the first trimester of pregnancy and two in the third trimester. No case occurred in labour, but of note for this chapter is that 10 deaths occurred after delivery at between 5 days and 4 weeks, indicating that labour was unlikely to be a risk factor. Seven of the bleeds were from aneurysm. In the other cases the source of bleeding was unknown.

SAH, although rare, is associated with poor outcome, with a general population-based case fatality rate of around 40% (van Gijn 1997). A literature review of cerebrovascular pathology during pregnancy and postpartum found a mean incidence of SAH of 20 per 100,000 deliveries. This is about five times greater than outside parturition, although the reviewers noted methodological weaknesses in some of the studies (Lamy et al 1996). It is suggested that the haemodynamic, hormonal or other physiological changes of pregnancy may play a role in increasing the likelihood of aneurysmal rupture (Lamy et al 1996).

A systematic review of risk factors for SAH in the general population was carried out, which included nine longitudinal studies and 11 case–control studies (Teunissen et al 1996). Smoking, hypertension and alcohol were found to be the most significant risk factors. No studies were identified, however, that had examined risk factors for SAH in postpartum populations, although among females generally neither oral contraceptive use nor HRT has shown any association.

## Management

Although this is a rare symptom, as over half of the deaths attributed to SAH during 2000–2002 reviewed by CEMACH (Lewis & Drife 2004) occurred more than 5 days after the birth, vigilance is required postpartum. With such a high case fatality rate, early referral of SAH to a specialist centre is essential. Diagnosis is usually confirmed using CT scan and lumbar puncture (Sztark et al 1996). On average, primary healthcare professionals will only encounter a patient with a SAH every 8 years (Linn et al 1996). It is likely that most healthcare professionals will never see a case in a postpartum woman, although women presenting with a sudden and violent or severe headache should be taken seriously and referred immediately.

## SUMMARY OF THE EVIDENCE USED IN THIS GUIDELINE

- Large observational studies have found that headaches are relatively common after childbirth, although there are no comparative studies of postpartum and non-postpartum women.
- Large observational studies have shown that PDPH can occur after spinal anaesthesia and trials have shown lower rates with smaller diameter and non-cutting needles.
- Although accidental puncture during epidural is uncommon, case series have shown that the incidence of PDPH after this is very high.
- Further studies, including randomised controlled trials, are required to assess the long-term effectiveness of treatments commonly used to *manage* symptoms of PDPH following epidural or spinal anaesthesia.
- Few studies have investigated the prevalence of *postpartum* hypertensive disorders.

- A systematic review including six small trials addressed the prevention and management of postpartum hypertension. There were no reliable data to guide management of women who are hypertensive postpartum or at increased risk of this symptom, and management decisions should be based on clinical judgement.
- Various types of descriptive studies of eclampsia have shown that this can be heralded by prodromal symptoms, although these may be of very short duration and in some cases, there may be an absence of symptoms prior to convulsion; 29–44% of all cases of eclampsia occur in the postnatal period.
- A systematic review including six trials of effectiveness of magnesium sulphate and other anticonvulsants for women with pre-eclampsia showed that use of magnesium sulphate with placebo or no anticonvulsant halved the risk of eclampsia.
- Two systematic reviews, one comparing magnesium sulphate with diazepam and one comparing magnesium sulphate with phenytoin, concluded that magnesium sulphate was substantially more effective in reducing the recurrence of convulsions
- Subarachnoid haemorrhage presenting with a sudden violent headache is extremely rare, but often fatal.

## WHAT TO DO

### Initial assessment

- All women should have a minimum of one BP measurement carried out and documented within 6 hours of giving birth (NICE 2006).
- All women should be advised of the signs and symptoms of pre-eclampsia/eclampsia and of the need to contact their healthcare professional immediately if they experience any of these (NICE 2006).
- Women should be asked about headache symptoms at each postnatal contact (NICE 2006).

The following questions should be posed in order to exclude possible diagnoses other than tension headache or migraine.

- Ask about the onset of the headache, the location and duration. Has the woman suffered any trauma to the head?
- If the woman had epidural/spinal analgesia, is the headache relieved by lying down?
- Ask about other conditions that produce, exacerbate or relieve the headache.
- Does the woman have a history of hypertension? (If hypertensive, see section below.)
- What degree of incapacity does the headache cause, i.e. can the woman carry out normal activities, do the headaches interfere with or prevent sleep?

**The symptoms listed below are not typical and appropriate referral should be made for assessment**

- Complaints of violent and sudden-onset ('thunderclap') headache, possibly with vomiting.
- Generalised headache where there is intense pain in the back of the neck or signs of fever.
- Headache associated with trauma.
- Progressively worsening headache.

**Symptoms suggestive of postpartum 'simple' headache (tension headache, or migraine)**

- If known migraine sufferer, continue with usual medication.
- If the woman has learnt relaxation techniques during the antenatal period she should be encouraged to continue these to relieve tension. If not, give advice on these.
- Discuss changes in childcare – explore ways to ensure sufficient sleep, e.g. relative/friend may care for the baby for a period during the day when the mother can rest.
- Mild analgesia can be advised – try paracetamol. If analgesia insufficient or further assessment required, the woman should be referred.
- Attempt to identify with the woman any factors which may trigger the headache, and ways in which these can be avoided.
- Reassure the woman that headaches are common and are generally no major cause for concern.

**Symptoms suggestive of PDPH**

- Where severe PDPH is suspected (especially if accidental dural puncture) referral should be made in accordance with local policy (urgent action). Some women may require hospital admission for assessment and treatment (blood patch).
- If the headache is severe, the woman should be encouraged to lie down and rest, to alleviate symptoms. Bed rest will not *prevent* headaches.
- Check and record blood pressure/temperature/pulse to obtain baseline.
- Where symptoms are moderate, should include simple analgesia advice in addition to reassurance.
- Bending or lifting should be avoided until the headache resolves.
- Hydration might help so check that fluid intake is adequate.
- Advise woman about possible diagnosis and that treatment is available.
- Ensure woman has available support to help her care for her infant and herself whilst she is experiencing the headaches.
- Visit as required to assess progress.

## Headache associated with hypertensive disorders

- Where a woman complains of headache in the postpartum period, has hypertension and there are other signs or symptoms of pre-eclampsia such as epigastric discomfort, visual disturbance, nausea or vomiting, NICE (2006) recommends immediate referral for further investigation (emergency action).
- If a woman's diastolic blood pressure is above 90 mmHg but she has no other signs or symptoms of pre-eclampsia, NICE (2006) recommends that the measurement is repeated within 4 hours; if the pressure has not fallen, she should be referred immediately for further investigation (emergency action).
- If a woman's diastolic blood pressure is above 90 mmHg and she has signs and symptoms of pre-eclampsia, NICE (2006) recommends that the woman is immediately referred for investigation (emergency action).
- If the woman complains of severe headache and has a history of hypertension in pregnancy, NICE (2006) recommends immediate referral (emergency action).
- Known essential hypertension is less worrying than a history of hypertension in pregnancy; continue management as medical instructions, ensure that the woman has appropriate follow-up. Immediate referral should be made if the woman has signs or symptoms of pre-eclampsia (see above).
- If hypertension is uncomplicated the woman should be reassured and simple analgesia given for the headache.
- In all the above cases review the woman the following day.
- Discuss any concerns about hypertensive disorders in a woman with the most appropriate healthcare professional at any time if indicated.

## General advice

- Provide information on signs and symptoms of pre-eclampsia.
- Avoid factors which precipitate or exacerbate headache.
- Take short rest periods when possible during the day.
- Do relaxation exercises.

# SUMMARY GUIDELINE

## Headache

### Initial assessment

To exclude diagnoses other than tension headache/migraine:

- Obtain baseline recording of BP (at least one BP measurement should be obtained within 6 hours of the birth)
- Ask about onset, location and duration of headache. History of trauma?

- Did the woman have epidural/spinal analgesia, and is headache postural (possible PDPH)?
- Are there other conditions which produce, exacerbate or relieve the headache?
- Is there a history of hypertension?
- What degree of incapacity does the headache produce?

## Emergency action is required if

- Diastolic BP ≥90 mmHg, with signs or symptoms of pre-eclampsia
- Diastolic BP remains ≥90 mmHg when repeated 4 hours after baseline in absence of signs or symptoms of pre-eclampsia
- Severe headache and history of hypertension during pregnancy
- Severe and sudden onset of 'thunderclap' headache
- Headache associated with trauma
- Headache associated with pyrexia, signs of fever
- Severe or persistent headaches

## What to do

### Postpartum 'Simple' headache

- If known migraine sufferer, continue with usual medication
- Advise on relaxation
- Discuss childcare and sleep – ways to have a rest during the day?
- Mild analgesia (paracetamol) can be advised. If analgesia insufficient refer (urgent action)
- Attempt to identify factors which trigger headache
- Reassure that headache is common and is generally no cause for concern

### Symptoms of PDPH

- Contact anaesthetic department at hospital where delivered
- Bed rest will alleviate symptoms but not prevent a headache
- Record BP, temperature and pulse
- Paracetamol can be taken as necessary
- Avoid bending/lifting until headache resolved
- Dehydration should be avoided
- Tell woman about possible diagnosis and that treatment is available
- Support with infant care
- Review as required

### Headaches and hypertensive disorders

- If diastolic BP is ≥90 mmHg, with signs and symptoms of pre-eclampsia, refer (emergency action)
- If diastolic BP is ≥90 mmHg but no signs and symptoms of pre-eclampsia, repeat measurement within 4 hours. If pressure has not fallen, refer (emergency action)
- Known hypertension – management as described, observe for symptoms of pre-eclampsia
- Review the next day in all cases
- Discuss hypertension with relevant healthcare professional at any time if indicated

## References

Atterbury J, Groome L, Hoff C et al 1998 Clinical presentation of women readmitted with postpartum severe preeclampsia or eclampsia. J Gynecol Neonatal Nurs 27(2): 134-141

Banks S, Paech M, Gurrin L 2001 An audit of epidural blood patch after accidental dural puncture with a Tuohy needle in obstetric patients. Int J Obstet Anaesth 10: 172-176

Barrett G 1996 Primary care for women: assessment and management of headache. J Nurse Midwif 41(2): 117-124.

Berger C, Crosby E, Grodecki W 1998 North American survey of the management of dural puncture occurring during labour epidural analgesia. Can J Anaesth 45(2): 110-114

Broughton Pipkin F 1995 Fortnightly review: the hypertensive disorders of pregnancy. BMJ 311: 609-613

Cesarini M, Torrielli R, Lahaye F et al 1990 Sprotte needle for intrathecal anaesthesia for Caesarean section: incidence of postdural puncture headache. Anaesthesia 45: 656-658

Chames M, Livingstone J, Thomas S et al 2002 Late postpartum eclampsia: a preventable disease? Am J Obstet Gynecol 186: 1174-1177

Chan T, Ahmed A, Yentis S et al 2003 Postpartum headaches: summary report of the National Obstetric Anaesthetic Database (NOAD) 1999. Int J Obstet Anaesth 12: 107-112

Choi A, Laurito C, Cunningham F 1996 Pharmacologic management of postdural puncture headache. Ann Pharmacol 30(7-8): 831-839

Cooper G 1999 Epidural blood patch. Editorial. Eur J Anaesth 16: 211-215

Crawford J 1972 The prevention of headache consequent upon dural puncture. Br J Anaesth 44: 598-600

Crawford J 1979 Experience with spinal analgesia in a British obstetric unit. Br J Anaesth 51: 531-535

Davey D, MacGillivray I 1988 The classification of the hypertensive disorders of pregnancy. Am J Obstet Gynecol 158(4): 892-898

Douglas K, Redman C 1994 Eclampsia in the United Kingdom. BMJ 309: 1359-1400

Duley L, Henderson-Smart D 2003b Magnesium sulphate versus diazepam for eclampsia. Cochrane Data Base of Systematic Reviews, Issue 4

Duley L, Henderson-Smart D 2003c Magnesium sulphate versus phenytoin for eclampsia. Cochrane Database of Systematic Reviews, Issue 4

Duley L, Gülmezoglu AM, Henderson-Smart DJ 2003a Magnesium sulphate and other anticonvulsants for women with pre-eclampsia. Cochrane Database of Systematic Reviews, Issue 2

Ferrazzani S, De Carolis S, Pomini F et al 1994 The duration of hypertension in the puerperium of preeclamptic women: relationship with renal impairment and week of delivery. Am J Obstet Gynecol 171(2): 506-512

Garcia J, Marchant S 1993 Back to normal? Postnatal health and illness. Paper presented at the Research and the Midwife Conference, University of Manchester

Gifford RW Jr, August PA, Cunningham G et al 2000 Report of the National High Blood Pressure Education Program Working Group on high blood pressure in pregnancy. Am J Obstet Gynecol 183(suppl):1-22

Glazener C, Abdalla M, Stroud P et al 1995 Postnatal maternal morbidity: extent, causes, prevention and treatment. Br J Obstet Gynaecol 102: 282-297

Gleeson C, Reynolds F 1998 Accidental dural puncture rates in UK obstetric practice. Int J Obstet Anaesth 7: 242-246

Grove L 1973 Backache, headache and bladder dysfunction after delivery. Br J Anaesth 45: 1147-1149

Gutsche B 1990 Lumbar epidural analgesia in obstetrics: taps and patches. In: Reynolds F (ed) Epidural and spinal blockade in obstetrics. Baillière Tindall, London

Halpern S, Preston R 1994 Postdural puncture headache and spinal needle design. Metaanalyses. Anesthesiology 81: 1376-1383

Hopkinson J, Samaan A, Russell I et al 1997 A comparative multicentre trial of spinal needles for Caesarean section. Anaesthesia 52(10): 1005-1011

Hughes D, Simmons SW, Brown J et al 2003 Combined spinal-epidural versus epidural analgesia in labour. Cochrane Database of Systematic Reviews, Issue 4

International Headache Society 2004 International classification of headache disorders. Cephalalgia 24(1)

Katz J, Aidinis S 1980 Current concepts review. Complications of spinal and epidural anesthesia. J Bone Joint Surg 62A(7): 1219-1222

Lamy C, Sharshar T, Mas J 1996 Cerebralvascular diseases in pregnancy and puerperium. Revue Neurologique 152(6-7): 422-440

Lewis G, Drife J (eds) 2004 Why mothers die 2000–2002. Report on Confidential Enquiries into Maternal Deaths in the United Kingdom. RCGP Press, London

Linn F, Rinkel G, Algra A et al 1996 Incidence of subarachnoid haemorrhage – role of region, year and rate of computed tomography: a meta-analysis. Stroke 27(14): 625-629

Lubarsky S, Barton J, Friedman S et al 1994 Late postpartum eclampsia revisited. Obstet Gynecol 83(4): 502-505

Lybecker H, Djernes M, Schmidt J 1995 Postdural puncture headache (PDPH): onset, duration, severity and associated symptoms. An analysis of 75 consecutive patients with PDPH. Acta Anaesthesiol Scand 39: 605-612

MacArthur C, Lewis M, Knox E 1991 Health after childbirth. HMSO, London

MacArthur C, Lewis M, Knox E 1993 Accidental dural puncture in obstetric patients and long term symptoms. BMJ 306: 883-885

MacArthur C, Winter H, Bick D et al 2003 Redesigning postnatal care: a randomised controlled trial of protocol based, midwifery led care focused on individual women's physical and psychological health needs. NHS R and D, NCC HTA

Madej T, Jackson I, Wheatley R et al 1993 Assessing introduction of spinal anaesthesia for obstetric procedures. Quality Health Care 2: 31-34

Magee L, Sadeghi S 2005 Prevention and treatment of postpartum hypertension. Cochrane Database of Systematic Reviews, Issue 1. Update Software, Oxford

McSwiney M, Phillips J 1995 Post dural puncture headache. Acta Anaesthesiol Scand 39: 990-995

Meher S, Duley L 2006 Rest during pregnancy for preventing pre-eclampsia and its complications in women with normal blood pressure. Cochrane Database of Systematic Reviews, Issue 2. Update Software, Oxford

National Institute for Health and Clinical Excellence (NICE) 2003 Antenatal care: routine care for the healthy pregnant woman. National Institute for Health and Clinical Excellence, London

National Institute for Health and Clinical Excellence (NICE) 2006 Postnatal care: routine postnatal care of women and their babies. National Institute for Health and Clinical Excellence, London

Ng K, Parsons J, Cyna AM et al 2004 Spinal versus epidural anaesthesia for caesarean section. Cochrane Database of Systematic Reviews, Issue 2. Update Software, Oxford

Pitt B 1973 'Maternity blues'. Br J Psychiatry 122: 431-433

Rasmussen B 1993 Migraine and tension-type headache in a general population: precipitating factors, female hormones, sleep pattern and relation to lifestyle. Pain 53: 65-72

Richman JM, Joe E, Cohen S et al 2006 Bevel direction and postdural puncture headache: a meta-analysis. Neurologist 12 (4): 224-228

Saurel-Cubizolles M-J, Romito P, Lelong N et al 2000 Women's health after childbirth: a longitudinal study in France and Italy. Br J Obstet Gynaecol 107: 1202-1209

Shutt L, Valentine S, Wee M et al 1992 Spinal anaesthesia for Caesarean section: comparison of 22 gauge and 25 gauge Whitacre needles with 26 gauge Quincke needles. Br J Anaesth 69: 589-594

Stein G 1981 Headaches in the first postpartum week and their relationship to migraine. Headache 21: 201-205

Stein G, Morton J, Marsh A et al 1984 Headaches after childbirth. Acta Neurol Scand 69: 74-79

Stride P, Cooper G 1993 Dural taps revisited. Anaesthesia 48: 247-255

Sudlow C, Warlow C 2001 Epidural blood patching for preventing and treating post-dural puncture headache. Cochrane Database of Systematic Reviews, Issue 2. Update Software, Oxford

Sztark F, Petitjean M, Thicoipe M et al 1996 Subarachnoid haemorrhage caused by aneurysm rupture. Initial management of patients. Ann Fr Anesth Reanim 15(3): 322-327

Taivainen T, Pitkanen M, Trominen M et al 1993 Efficacy of epidural blood patch for post-dural puncture headache. Acta Anaesthesiol Scand 37: 702-705

Tan LK, de Swiet M 2002 The management of postpartum hypertension. Br J Obstet Gynaecol 109 (7): 733-736

Teunissen L, Rinkel G, Algra A et al 1996 Risk factors for subarachnoid haemorrhage: a systematic review. Stroke 27(3): 544-549

Tufnell DJ, Jankowicz D, Lindow SW et al 2005 Outcomes of severe pre-eclampsia/eclampsia in Yorkshire 1999/2003. Br J Obstet Gynaecol 112(7): 875-880

Turnbull D K, Shepherd D B 2003 Post-dural puncture headache: pathogenesis, prevention and treatment. British Journal of Anaesthesia; 91(5): 718-729.

van Gijn J 1997 Slip-ups in diagnosis of subarachnoid haemorrhage. Lancet 349: 1492

Vandam L, Dripps R 1956 Long term follow up of patients who received 10098 spinal anaesthetics. JAMA 161: 586-591

Walters B, Thompson M, Lee A et al 1986 Blood pressure in the puerperium. Clin Sci 71(5): 589-594

Wasserberg J, Barlow P 1997 Lumbar puncture still has an important role in diagnosing subarachnoid haemorrhage. BMJ 315: 1598-1599

# Appendices

# Appendix 1

# Search strategy for second edition

Searches of the literature were conducted to update the postnatal care evidence base from the years 2000 to 2006. A systematic review of common health problems during the postnatal period was conducted for the *Postnatal Care Guideline* published by NICE in July 2006.[1] The synthesis of the literature which underpins the guideline recommendations has been used as the primary basis for the update of this book.

The search strategy for the guideline included an initial review of published guidelines or systematic reviews using a wide range of databases and websites, including National Electronic Library for Health (NeLH) Guidelines Finder, National Guidelines Clearinghouse, Scottish Intercollegiate Guidelines Network (SIGN), Guidelines International Network (GIN), Canadian Medical Association (CMA) Infobase (Canadian guidelines), National Health and Medical Research Council (NHMRC) Clinical Practice Guidelines (Australian Guidelines), New Zealand Guidelines Group, BMJ Clinical Evidence, MIDIRS (Midwives Information & Resource Service), Cochrane Database of Systematic Reviews (CDSR), Database of Abstracts of Reviews of Effects (DARE) and Heath Technology Assessment Database (HTA).

Further searching for the guideline was carried out by topic, using all or some of the following bibliographic databases which were searched from their inception to the latest date available: MEDLINE, EMBASE, CINAHL, CENTRAL (Cochrane Controlled Trials Register), PsycINFO, Allied & Complementary Medicine (AMED), DH-Data (Department of Health) & British Nursing Index (BNI).

The highest level of evidence was sought by the guideline developers. Observational studies, surveys and expert formal consensus results were used only when randomised control trials were not available and in many cases they were not. Only English language papers were reviewed.

---

[1] DeMott K, Bick D, Norman R, Ritchie G, Turnbull N, Adams C, Barry C, Byrom S, Elliman D, Marchant S, McCandlish R, Mellows H, Neale C, Parkar M, Tait P, Taylor C, (2006) *Clinical Guidelines and Evidence Review for Post natal care: Routine post natal care of recently delivered women and their babies* London: National Collaborating Centre for Primary Care and Royal College of General Practitioners).

A final update search for this edition of *Postnatal Care* was carried out in summer 2006 to identify any further additions to the evidence base specifically for prevalence and risk factors. Some studies published since then are included but not based on a systematic search. These searches were intentionally broad topical searches (see example below) carried out to identify all potentially relevant studies. The following bibliographic databases were searched from the year 2000 to the latest date available: MEDLINE, EMBASE, MIDIRS (including relevant CINAHL entries), CENTRAL (Cochrane Controlled Trials Register) and DARE.

Example: search strategy for perineal pain, risk incidence

| # | Search History |
|---|---|
| 1 | postnatal care.mp. |
| 4 | postpartum period.mp. |
| 5 | (postpartum or puerpera$ or puerperium).tw. |
| 6 | (new mother or first time mother$).tw. |
| 7 | puerpera$.tw. |
| 8 | (postnatal period$ or postnatal care).tw. |
| 9 | (post delivery or postdelivery).tw. |
| 10 | (post birth or postbirth).tw. |
| 11 | (multipara$ or primipara$ or nullipara$).tw. |
| 13 | perineal pain.mp. [mp=ti, ab, sh, hw, tn, ot, dm, mf, nm] |
| 14 | perin$ pain.tw. |
| 17 | (risk factor or prevalence or incidence).tw. |

# Appendix 2

# Symptom checklist

I am going to ask if you have experienced any of the following health problems since having your baby. These are all health problems which many women experience after childbirth. If we know you have a particular problem, we may be able to offer advice or treatment to help it.

Since having your baby, have you experienced:

| | Guideline No. | Date | | Date | |
|---|---|---|---|---|---|
| | | YES | NO | YES | NO |
| Abnormal bleeding | 1 | | | | |
| Perineal pain or dyspareunia | 2 | | | | |
| Abdominal wound problems | 3 | | | | |
| Breastfeeding problems | 4 | | | | |
| Urinary problems (ask about stress incontinence, UTI, voiding difficulties) | 5 | | | | |
| Bowel problems (ask about constipation, haemorrhoids, loss of control) | 6 | | | | |
| Depression | 7 | | | | |
| Fatigue | 8 | | | | |
| Backache | 9 | | | | |
| Headache | 10 | | | | |

PLEASE REFER TO APPROPRIATE GUIDELINE FOR SUGGESTED MANAGEMENT OF EACH SYMPTOM IDENTIFIED

# Subject index

Notes, Page numbers in *italics* refer to figures and those in **bold** denote tables